Gorgeous!

How to look
and feel
fantastic
every day

Adele Stickland

Gorgeous!

First published in 2019 by

Panoma Press Ltd
48 St Vincent Drive, St Albans, Herts, AL1 5SJ, UK
info@panomapress.com
www.panomapress.com

Book layout by Neil Coe.

Printed on acid-free paper from managed forests.

ISBN 978-1-784521-60-8

Dedication

To all gorgeous girls

Testimonials

"Adele's enthusiasm, extensive knowledge and ability to inspire change leap off every page – a really good read."

Sally Jackson, reversing type 2 diabetes coach and Arbonne consultant, RGN, EdD

"You cannot fail to be motivated and inspired by Adele's infectious enthusiasm and holistic approach."

Dr Penny McCarthy BSc (Hons), BMedSci, BMBS, DRCOG, MRCGP

"A great book from Adele about the 'whys' and 'hows' of self-care, so much good advice with the science and references to back it up."

Dr Kate Thomas MBBS, MRCGP (retired GP)

"Educational, insightful and funny."

Jo, mum of two

"Compelling read that dispels the myths of dieting and gives you the lifelong tools to step into your Gorgeousness."

Sandra, business owner

"Thoughtful, practical and actionable advice to ensure the weight you lose this time will stay off for good."

Julie Dennis, menopause coach and trainer

"Adele's insights and enthusiasm leap off the page and inspire positive change."

Trina Lake, journalist

Acknowledgements

To the amazing women I have met on my own gorgeous journey including and especially my 'mam', sisters, bro, fabulous Dave, who swims like a fish, and to my wonderful kids – thank you.

Contents

Introduction

Get Gorgeous is an online group of women interested in healthy eating and sustainable weight loss. I set it up in 2015 to help stressed-out career women and professional mums. Having worked in the fitness and wellness industry for over 20 years, and with a personal fertility issue that spanned 10 years, I developed a drive for health and wellbeing that became a personal obsession.

The more I worked with women, the more upset and troubled I became about clearing up their diet myths. I spoke to shocked women who had followed 'diet guidelines' for half their lives, only to find out that despite 'not having a sweet tooth' they had ended up with diabetes. The lack of understanding that carbohydrates or 'carbs' (all carbs) break down into glucose (sugar) in your body, whether it is a slice of rye from handsome Pete at the organic grocery shop or a packet of biscuits, plagued me. Why don't women know this?

Your body will use the glucose (from carbs) before it even begins to use fat in your love handles as fuel. Vegetables contain carbs, fruit contains carbs and biscuits contain carbs, as do bread, oats and bananas. With headlines that scream "fats are bad" and "eating too much protein is bad for you", it is not surprising that most women are confused. Nutrition has become sensationalised – tabloid headlines are our daily digestive intake. It is time for a commonsensical, down to earth and factual approach.

With the misconceptions of the healthy heart diet and the population's current high-carb predisposition, your diet is anything but balanced. Going back to basics and examining the ratio of your macronutrients – your carbs, proteins and fats – is your first step. Don't worry about what milk to put in your tea – almond, cow's or soya. That is introspective and too detailed. Instead, take the time to assess the bigger 'macro' picture of what you are eating every day.

Mismanaging macros is the first myth-busting concept this book will tackle and challenging the diet industry will be the second objective. Looking at why this has happened and how you can get out of your own way are also core objectives.

Diet yo-yoing is dangerous, but why? Why are diets so dangerous to the female body? Visit my Get Gorgeous website (www.get-gorgeous.com) and you'll find my free ebook explaining why diets simply don't work.

It is not down to your lack of willpower or laziness. When you fixate on the food you are not allowed, that food becomes harder to resist. Neurologically your brain is being forced into a negative cycle of deprivation. This book will talk at length about your inner teenager and how she is very uncomfortable about being told what to do. I have worked with hundreds of clients who have pet names for their inner teenagers; they are varied and amusing. By the end of the book you will have your own personal, inner teenager to work with.

The simple truth is that women's bodies have an invested, biological reason to hold on to fat. Fat is a precious resource for your brain and every one of your cells. Your body is not going to waste that resource. As soon as the female body experiences hunger over a prolonged period, it will shut down its non-essential functions. Metabolic changes happen in your body when you go without food and your metabolism slows. Your body moves into 'starvation' mode and stops you burning fat and calories. Your body finds a way to run itself on fewer calories. [1]

Diets don't work.

The diet industry is exactly that – an industry. It produces healthy-looking products which use clean-looking typefaces, images and wording that dupe you and me into thinking the product is going to help our energy levels and bum size. I've consumed green smoothies – the packaging and ingredients looked amazing, but wait a minute, when was this 'product' processed? What has gone into it to give it a 'healthy' shelf life?

Like a little ear worm, I am going to change your life. You can continue with your normal routine, and this book and my online resources will help you to add in a few, easy habits that will change your thinking about food. Slowly and over time you will look and feel fantastic every day!

This book will slowly tease open your mind, plant a few new thoughts and ultimately change the direction of your life. You will lose weight. I'm going to hypnotise you into it; my little voice will be with you now for the rest of your life. You can argue with me, by all means, you can shout at me and laugh with me. But I *will* change your preconceptions and I *will* be the nagging, challenging conceptions voice for years to come.

The first few chapters begin with pushing the 'good girl' mindset off the school bench. Good girl syndrome, as I have coined it, is that feeling that you must be seen as perfect, working hard and never rocking the boat. Then spoon in a big dollop of an "I am worthy because I'm so hard-working" mindset. That needy, working hard, victim mentality is in all women, me included. I am going to dislodge that badge of honour; it may not come off straight away, but you will become aware of how you talk to yourself.

Katie and I brought up our firstborn sons together. She is my oldest BFF [best friend forever] and she laughs when we chat, "You are not a witch... exactly... Adele." She never quite finishes that sentence. I will talk you round, cajole, interest, make you laugh and annoy you all in the space of one book. You can tick those emotions off as you go through.

Chapter 1 is about knowing yourself. Find out how you operate, what your triggers are and how you can get out of your own way. Chapter 2 moves forward and gives your 'mindset frog' a push off the lily pad – in a way that reassures you and helps you move forward, explaining that everything is going to be OK for you. Your self-awareness and confidence will grow.

You'll discover my big sister tendencies in Chapter 3 as I move you through and beyond your negative, self-sabotaging talk, explaining why it is imperative that you smile through adversity and look for the positive in life. An overexuberant, happy demeanour may be irritating, but scientists have established that once you take a positive approach to life you will be happier and feel fantastic in the longer term.

No more "life's not fair", because you will miss out on opportunities and gifts: this is explored in Chapter 3. Chapter 4 explores your guiding spirit, who she is and how she can help guide your life, your health and your weight loss. Ensuring that you take care of yourself is an essential part of female growth and has been sadly lacking over the last 2,000 years. Chapter 5 outlines why caring for yourself is your duty.

The second part of the book becomes a little racier, moves a little faster and illustrates why you do have a perfect weight and the nutritional science behind it. Chapter 6 explains how easy it is to obtain your perfect size once you have come to terms with and accepted who you are. Mental health is an intrinsic part of your health, the first step to true grace, dignity and beauty now and later in life – this is covered in Chapter 7. Chapter 8 outlines that basic movement is an essential part of your health, and is very different from a brisk walk in the park or three times a week at the gym. That is simply not enough to win the war on your health. Your posture is paramount to your bone health, muscle strength, and overall sexiness. As a posture bore, I will outline great posture, perfect balance, optimum strength and how you need to move more and exercise less, in the last chapter.

This book will help you to navigate past sensational diet headlines and offer you the opportunity to examine the science in an open and 'digestible' way. You will have the knowledge and references to make up your own mind. Weight loss in your 40s and 50s is easy. I've done it, the gorgeous girls have done it. This book will show you how we have achieved it.

Have fun and please feel free to shout out loud at me as you read this book. Feel free to post your comments on my blogs, vlogs and Facebook pages. Let's start a conversation, let's bring women's health and self-esteem out in the open.

Chapter notes

I should note that I have been living in Devon for nearly 15 years and in Devon every inanimate object is given a gender. It is incredibly endearing. With intent on humour, I shall carry on with this time-honoured tradition and even extend it to imply that everything that is wrong is a 'he' and everything that is goddess-like and wonderful is a 'she'. It is a joke, it is fun, so don't get offended. Throughout the book, I shall discuss 'Rule Number 7', which was introduced to me by my daughter's violin teacher: "Don't take life too seriously." You will discover this in the forthcoming chapters as doors open and your eyes widen.

This is a book of devotion and love to you the reader. I want you to be the gorgeous girl you have always meant to be. Headspace that is filled with negativity does not help you or your loved ones. I want you to shine and be gloriously gorgeous. I want you to look and feel and fantastic every day!

*"The World will be saved by
the western woman."*

The Dalai Lama, at the Vancouver Peace Summit 2009

CHAPTER 1

You must get out of your own way

Most people aren't aware that they are in their own way, let alone being able to decide how to get out of it. Perhaps you are completely unaware that you have 'done what your parents expected', or simply followed the natural route that you felt was available to you. I followed a law degree path because it sounded like a professional option, only to find out halfway through that I was not meant to be a lawyer. After university, I worked in marketing, starting with a temp job with Saatchi & Saatchi in Edinburgh, simply because I thought advertising sounded cool. For eight years I followed that path, until Ben, our son, had other ideas.

Neither of these paths ended up being my chosen one, the one that brings me to chat to you today. They informed me and shaped the person that I am today, but they were not my passion, my flow in life.

The point I am making is: who makes your life decisions? What has brought you to this point in your life right now? What life decisions have you made based on life flow rather than purposeful decisions? Do you recognise your anchor points, the times or points in time that changed your life and its direction?

Crashing and burning out of corporate life when my first son was born forced a change in my life. When were your big, right-hand turns? Perhaps your changes have come about because of dramatic, life-changing circumstance, or perhaps you have planned your life in a systematic way?

Whether your life has been in flow or you have deliberately organised it, there will be underlining, beneath the surface emotional currents or predispositions that have affected your choices. Familial expectations may have affected your life choices. Did you become an architect, marketer, GP, lawyer, corporate high-flyer or small business success because it was expected of you? Are you aware of your ancestral and emotional line and how it has affected your choices in life?

Unlock your past

Perhaps, like me, you came from a poor background and the only personal growth option you felt available to you was university. My 'mam' came from the Gorbals, the slums of Glasgow, which have since been demolished. The only way out was education. That was my early subliminal learning. In his youth, my dad played in the rubble of the bomb sites of London. He never went to university and although he was extremely well read and eloquent, his life motto from the 1960s was, "Let it all hang out." I therefore inherited a tendency to speak up, which offers an interesting juxtaposition at times.

Other family messages in my life and yours are food-orientated. For instance, my mum had three brothers and was the only daughter. It was a race for her to finish her food before her starving brothers started eating hers. She had to eat quickly and yet was always the last to be served. The subliminal message for her was that "the working man needed his food first".

As a result of my mum's pain, I was always given the same amount of food on my plate as my dad.

Caroline was also motivated to finish everything on her plate and have seconds. Her father, an American, was brought up in the American Depression before the 1950s white bread era.[1] He experienced a severe feeling of scarcity; meals always had seconds and most of the time, thirds.

The Irish potato famine is a distant memory from three generations ago, and yet the feeling of 'going without' remains. Considering food to be a scarcity and feeling famished is still part of an ancestral line. Rationing during and after the second world war (the original 'clean' eating in the UK [2] has left an ancestral pattern in many people's lives. We have messages that follow us and work with us now in our daily lives. You may not be aware of all these messages, but you will be aware of your behaviour – which stems from these messages.

Part of getting out of your own way is knowing how you respond to life's emotional see-saw, who you really are and where your thought patterns come from. It is worth spending time observing whether these thoughts are serving you now, pondering whether your real emotional needs are being met, and even acknowledging whether you know what your needs are. What has been left unexplored and unnoticed? Left unexplored, these emotions and suppressed feelings affect the way you treat yourself. The only true person who can understand your needs is you.

Unlock your passion

Listening to your body, acknowledging how you feel will uncover bigger questions, such as what your motivations are in life and what really drives your passion. This thinking will help you to uncover your motivation. My first call with new clients is spent finding out their real passion in life, because that is what drives your quest for great health. Focusing on what will motivate you in the long term can allow you to get out of your own way and help you to uncover and circumvent old feelings and historical myths – for example, that food is scarce.

Linda was driven by work. On our first call, we discovered that her driving passion was her business. She was in an exciting, developmental stage of a new, personal business, having 'served' in the corporate world for decades. Linda's big vision for her business was creating a negative impact on her health. After much discussion and reflection, she realised that if her health wasn't working for her then she wouldn't have the clarity and stamina required to get the business up and running. It would fail if she didn't have her health to keep up the momentum. As soon as Linda and I connected her health choices to the drive forward in her business, the rest was easy.

Linda's passion for helping corporate executives to be more sustainable and create strong eco credentials in corporate big business was her driving force. Combining that with her own health meant we had the key to unlock her desire to be healthy for herself. Eating well and forgoing endless cups of coffee with sugar bombs was easy once Linda had aligned her business 'why' with her personal 'why'. Linda had to be performing at a top level to achieve her business dreams.

When you approach your health journey with an understanding that there is so much more below the surface, you realise that your everyday actions are the clues to unlocking your behaviours and, most importantly, your eating behaviours. Then finding your way forward with your personal motivational key is easy. When you accept, appreciate and understand yourself, finding your perfect healthy weight is easy to achieve.

It is not all about eating right and getting some fresh air, although that is enormously helpful. Sometimes your health journey starts with you, finding out where your 'head is at' or where your thoughts are and unblocking your routine, set behaviours.

Knowing yourself is the key to future success

Knowing yourself is the key to weight loss and healthy success. And success has a structure that includes your vision and goals. "Above all be true to yourself and know thyself" (paraphrased Shakespeare), or as often attributed to Oscar Wilde, "Be yourself. everyone else is already taken." Taking time to understand yourself will help you find the right course of action for you.

If you are looking for Insta-results, which are results-driven and as fast as your food,[3] you are missing your personal link between your subconscious thoughts and your behaviour: the reason why you behave as you do, the connection between your deep thoughts and your behaviour.

It could be as simple as eating everything on your plate because of your parents' wartime shortage or because your mum gives you more food than you need, because she missed out, as discussed previously.

You are aware that love can be inappropriately expressed through food. You know your loving and caring Aunt Flo will offer you sandwiches, cakes and biscuits simply because she is pleased to see you. How many times do you do this to yourself?

Knowing yourself is an interesting and thoughtful journey, which will offer you so much more than simply your weight loss. You are fascinating, you are intriguing, you are gorgeous.

Instant results don't work in the long term

A 'diet' action plan that gives no thought to what ultimately and truly motivates you will fail. Diets fail. You will end up back at square one if you are not aware of your own agenda. A personalised approach to your weight loss is your long-term key. Looking to know who you are, your triggers, what works for you and trusting your gorgeous body is your only true, sustainable way forward.

Some of your triggers are easy to spot and you will hear yourself repeat "I know, I know."

"I know I should be eating my veg, more protein, exercising more."

Be mindful that repeating, "I know, I know." is a mental shortcut that enables you to shut off your brain, to stop thinking about the barrage of information you receive and then avoid action.

Robert Cialdini[4] talks about mental shortcuts and how they are used every day to protect ourselves from information saturation. We create mental shortcuts and we become blind to our own behaviour. Some habitual behaviours become so ingrained and routine that we can miss them entirely. Ask yourself, "Why did I say that? What was my trigger when I reached for the biscuit in the meeting? Was it simply the only thing available and I am starving, or did I feel uncomfortable by what was being said and I needed a distraction?" Asking yourself questions will help you to think again about some of the actions that you have taken for granted.

Why do you diet?

Lifelong dieting. Isn't the clue in the word 'lifelong'? Recently I was chatting at a networking event to Kim and Sue, who had decided to go back on a diet. Kim was going back to the cabbage diet and Sue was going back to adding aspartame to her food to make it palatable so she could diet again. Shocking and yet predictable.

Diets are often habits and can even become a security blanket. They are a crutch for some people, despite the knowledge that they are affecting the delicate hormone balance of their body. As we age gracefully and approach the menopause, our hormones are more susceptible to the chemical changes that occur when we diet. Knowing yourself helps to understand your ability to change your behaviour, which can be critical around the menopause.

EXERCISE

Pause for a moment during your day and think, "Why do I do that?"

"What triggered my reaction to that abrupt receptionist?"

"What was I looking for when I drank that coffee: energy?"

"What really gives me the slight edge in a four-hour meeting?"

Are you open to growth?

Do you have a growth mindset? Are you open to change and new ideas? Are you ready to invest time in yourself and find out how you tick? Sally had a fixed mindset: "I always end up back at square one." She never managed to stick to diets and she was fearful and discouraged by past setbacks and failures.

"I have always been a big girl, I can't run, I am not made for running. I've never been able to stick at anything." Sally's phrases were being picked up by her subconscious and they steered her future. She was affirming who she was daily: big-boned, useless at exercise, never able to complete things. As a result, her subconscious couldn't believe that she could move on and change.

If your mindset is fixed, you don't believe you have the ability to change and be successful. You create a fixed way of thinking, a way of thinking that is self-fulfilling and self-perpetuating, and becomes a personalised 'neurosignature'. A neurosignature is a habitual way of thinking, like a brain groove, a needle stuck on a vinyl record, a repetitive thought or mindset that is on rinse and repeat. I will talk a lot about your neurosignature and how you can first be aware of your pattern, pause and create change.

When these thoughts are left uncovered and unquestioned, you create a pathway that you are used to listening to and working with. You carry a belief system around that prevents you from moving forward with your true life goal.

"The belief that your qualities are carved in stone leads to a host of thoughts and actions ..."

Carol Dweck [5]

If you are on a fragile footing and then use all your willpower to force a change that includes a diet of deprivation, you will fail. Without noticing what your true belief systems are a simple setback like a perceived criticism from a loved one can send you (and Sally) straight back to a downward spiral of "Why bother?" and reaching for comfort food.

Your brain can change and your brain signature can adapt, just as Sally's has. She learned to listen to her thoughts and call them out. She began to understand that they were not serving her. Sally did her due diligence, listened to her thoughts and associated her thoughts with a name from childhood. She learned to recognise when the childhood name was talking and she learned to reassure her childhood critic. Sally explained to her critic that it was OK and she may as well go outside and sunbathe. Sally was then able to move forward and create a strong, positive mindset. She found happiness and strength in her new gorgeous outlook and body. Sally moved forward in her life with a growth mindset and left her fixed mindset outside, sunbathing.

A growth mindset can be acquired easily

Your emotional intelligence can grow, your persistence in the face of obstacles can be nourished, and you can start feeling that you can learn from criticism rather than being diminished and feeling threatened by it. Having a growth mindset means you will thrive even during some of the challenging times of your life.

A growth mindset stretches you. Asking yourself questions creates a powerful passion for learning. Simply allowing and accepting growth will give you new paths.

Set your intention to grow and believe in yourself and that in itself will help you to overcome obstacles. Shifting your deep belief about yourself will guide your positive future outcomes and is the core message of this book.

Your inner dialogue is exhausting

Explore your own child critic, the inner dialogue that can keep you safe. She does go on a bit and listening to her is so tiring. As a child, your inner dialogue will tell you off if you are not behaving the way you 'should'. You can recognise your own 'perfect girl' syndrome: the perfect girl is very caring, looks after others and does a good job of keeping you safe.

Your perfect girl, inner critic has constant dialogue with you; she is working hard to keep you within your limited comfort zone, feeling secure. When you created her, however, you didn't have much life experience.

She tends to look for the mode of behaviour that will give you acceptance and gain love by those around you. [6] Your inner critic might be harsh and beat you up when you 'fail' to live up to your idealised, perfection goal. Stepping on those dreaded scales is a black and white reminder of your lost perfection. Inner critics are created to keep you safe and small when you are young. Instead, branch out and grow.

Call out and name your inner dementor

Anna calls her inner dementor 'Horace', (Harry Potter reference intended), which she feels is an appropriate name for her childhood critic. Naming her in this way helped Anna to identify when she was talking and where her mind chatter came from; Anna could decide if she wanted to listen to her 'Horace'.

Sally, from the previous example, used to ask 'Rose' – her childhood inner critic – to go and sit outside on a deckchair and tell her gently that it was OK and that she could handle this challenge now.

Perhaps you are so used to hearing and living with your inner critic that you don't even notice her anymore?

Monkey brain, inner chatter: they all add up to the same thing, which is inner doubt and lack of confidence, and your self-critic about food can have a lot to say. Listen for your inner critic and be aware of how you speak to yourself. You would have to have nerves of steel to put up with this barrage:

"I have always been fat, you fat cow, you shouldn't have eaten that – you are a failure"

"You will never get this right, you will never be skinny, why didn't you get out of bed this morning at 6am and start the couch to 5k?"

"What is wrong with me? Why am I so stupid? I can't learn anything"

"I have no time, I am too busy looking after XYZ."

Airing these thoughts and hearing them out in the open will extinguish the grip of Horace and Rose. Name your thoughts and your emotions. Deliberately and consciously speak your inner critic comments out loud; talk yourself through it and that will start the process of freeing your subconscious programming. Speaking out loud, journaling or talking to a coach like me will take something that is on autopilot with simmering anxiety and give you an insight into what is going on in your background.

By listening to your thoughts, you are making them come through into your conscious mind. That simple awareness formula will help to make the breakthrough and understand why you have stayed stuck in a particular diet cycle or even deeper, more destructive cycles of behaviour.

EXERCISE

Who is your critical voice and what does she say? What is her name?

Label and notice your critic with a catchy name like Felicity or there goes Prudence again or Horace or Rose is really going hell for leather today. Then you can begin to remove her from the scene, picture her voice receding into space or add a cartoon character to her voice and imagine that you can turn the volume down. Look for the humour in her comments and her voice.

You should never, ever argue with your inner dementor. She is way too clever, she will simply get louder and stamp her teenage foot. Smile nicely, acknowledge Horace or Rose and let her know that you have it covered, "Thanks, I've got this."

EXERCISE

Finish these sentences and listen to your responses with an interested ear:

"I always…"

"I never…"

"I am always…"

"I am never…"

Tune into your emotions

Between 5% and 10% of your mind is conscious and analytical. The decision-making part of your brain, where your judgment and evaluation come from, is your short-term working memory.

You don't know your thoughts, as around 95% of your mind is automated. Your thoughts can number as many as 20,000 to 70,000 a day.[7] If you name those thoughts, out loud, then you will make them conscious.

That is a huge number of comments to sift through. Here is an easier, more simplified way of analysing your thoughts: simply look for the emotion. If that conscious thought makes you 'feel uncomfortable', be guided by that feeling. When you recognise that uncomfortable, niggling pattern of thinking, you have the opportunity to review it. You have the opportunity to challenge your thinking and make a different choice, asking your vision or your higher self to take you in a new direction.

When you stop for a moment and listen to yourself speak in a disparaging way, you have the opportunity to consider making a change. Your brain will recognise that it has a chance and the ability to look for solutions to find an alternative.

Look at the energy flow in your body

When you speak, notice the feelings that you are hiding and watch the pattern of your behaviour. You may notice that your discomfort manifests itself in your eating and drinking habits, your moods and even your work strategy.

"Insight is the ability to see with with the eyes of the heart."

Michael Brown [8]

Your pause creates an opening

Just a moment's thought and awareness will give your brain a habit interruption strategy and creates the opportunity and choice to opt for a new course of action. It is as simple as making a momentary pause, which creates awareness and a new path for you.

Knowing that you have the choice and therefore the control is empowering and will effect a change that will alter the course of your life. Start small: simply listen to your thoughts, speak them out loud once in a while, notice them and air them. Be aware of your emotions and notice when you have 'triggered' an unrequited emotional experience. You will gradually learn to let the emotions go.

Love your sexy, big bum

Working with a mantra to replace these negative thoughts is wonderful tool. "I love myself" comes from Kamal Ravikant.[9] The divinity within you, your higher self, your inner mentor attracts a happier life to you. When speaking to yourself and others, choose whether you want to use words like 'heal', 'inspire', 'praise', 'encourage' and 'strength' rather than 'wound', 'criticise', 'discourage' or 'weakness'. Changing the way you speak to yourself will help you to achieve the goals and aspirations that you have always wanted.

Weight gain is the effect of un-interrogated emotions

Weight gain is the result of unmanaged, disturbing thoughts, overeating to compensate for feelings of hurt or eating because you deserve a treat and feel exhausted. Your ignorance of your emotional 'dis-ease' and discomfort will manifest through hurt, fright, pain or lack of personal care because of little or no self-management. Your weight is not the effect of your anguish: weight gain is caused by you ignoring your anguish. Suppressing your emotions leads to comfort eating.

Perceiving weight gain as the problem is the wrong way around. Your weight gain is simply a symptom of a bigger feeling of being uncomfortable. Emotional eating happens because of feeling uncomfortable in your body and your weight gain is the symptom.

When you feel uncomfortable, you tend to do something physical, such as changing your job, your home or even your partner. Comfort eating, drinking or moaning about how life is unfair are symptoms of a great unease in your body and your mind. Instead, pause and change the pattern and look within, exploring any discomfort that you may be feeling in your emotional body.

'Imprinting' describes the issue of emotions being passed down from your ancestors, or subliminal messages from your parents being internalised, as explored earlier. Interestingly, the 'good girl' bias that we all have is simply conditioning from authority figures, society and culture, which has been passed down to you.

Be present with your thoughts

When working one-to-one with clients, I love to dive into where emotions have been left and stranded in their body. All hurt, all pain is kept in your body. I am aware of that because of my physical training. It is easy to see how hunched shoulders are created through physical stresses or, more often, through emotional stress. Body pain isn't always in the easy-to-spot places like hunched shoulders: for me, my neck is my tension pain point. What is yours?

Being present with your thoughts gives you an opportunity to explore unwanted experiences stranded in your body. Being aware of your emotions will release them and create a new alignment and flow. If you are lost in your thoughts and feel anguish, then becoming present in your body is the most direct way back to your feelings.

This is why we eat emotionally: everyone does it to an extent. We all 'treat' ourselves. It is a permissible and enjoyable way to love life. Life should be made up of 'little gifts', but you don't have to take them all as food treats. Let's explore the other ways you can gift yourself when you feel sad, ashamed, unhappy or tired.

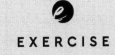

EXERCISE

How can you gift yourself?

Avoid blaming someone else

The frame of mind that it is someone else's fault distances you from your inner mentor. It creates a rift and a vacuum. The blame frame is the earnest belief that somebody else has created a feeling within you.

In the case of an argument with a neighbour or a spouse, for example, the onus is on you to accept responsibility and then you are free to solve the situation rather than holding a grudge until they apologise.

The blame frame doesn't have to be based on arguments. There are other variations, such as believing that your husband won't support you, that the kids need crisps in the house, or that there was nobody to go swimming or to Pilates with.

These beliefs, which feel very real, are superficial, the tip of the iceberg and prevent you from seeing below the surface. Blame is a symptom and the excuse that we hide behind to prevent change. Everybody does it. The gift of noticing how quickly you can own the situation and change it will help you to get on with your gorgeous life.

Often, what we receive is what we desire for others. What you think about you bring about is the simple law of attraction. The ancient Hindi word 'Genshai' means never treat another person, or yourself, in a manner that makes one feel small. [10]

Patterns of eating – genetics or programming?

There are many clues to our unconscious behaviour and once you shine the light of awareness on your own behaviour it is easier to identify and release these old behaviour patterns. For instance, insightful Gretchen Rubin [11] describes people as having one of four personality types: obligers, rebels, upholders and questioners. Which one of these personality types resonates with you?

Women generally fall into the obligers group. Obligers love to follow rules. Most of us are obligers, for whom seeking approval is a great motivator, even more than personal results. Which leads to an interesting trap of valuing other people's opinions more than our own.

For example, if your boss asks you to complete a report for tomorrow's meeting you may moan, groan and say how unfair or how unrealistic it is, but it will weigh you down and eventually you will get up at 5am or stay up to 11pm and get it done. You can't help yourself. Your 'good girl' programming kicks in.

Here is another scenario. You are mega busy, uber busy and you want to fit in your Pilates class, but your boss wants a report for tomorrow morning or Johnny says he needs trousers sewn up. What would you do? Would give up your personal agenda and follow Johnny's or your boss's? Of course you would. That is your societal programming around the belief that you would be seen as a bad employee, wife or mother.

If you follow this pattern, you are an obliger. You uphold the rules. You are kind, compassionate and above all a people pleaser. Obligers usually need an external form of accountability to get things done and that is why in the first instance diets will work for you. You are upholding somebody else's rules and regulations – until the inner teenager stamps her foot and doesn't take it anymore.

Upholders, on the other hand, follow their own rules and others (they are knackered most of the time because there are a lot of rules). Questioners debate the rules (rare and the more thoughtful and perhaps the less stressed personality type there is – unless, of course, they ask too many questions and they end up never getting started with anything). The final category are the rebels who are rare and speak for themselves. They don't *ever* follow the rules. They find a role in the military or the government so that they can rebel against the rules.

Our oldest son is a rebel, who rebelled against my 'education is the only way out' programming. I pushed him through education, working with his schoolteachers and organising extra tuition for his 11+ with a formidable ex-army education enforcer. He went through the motions, but when asked point blank whether he actually wanted to go to a grammar school he simply shouted back, "No!" Finally, I got the message.

He argued against university debt and societal programming, believing that self-worth doesn't have to come from a university education. He bucked the trend, and his aim to work hard in a career abroad, so that his references would be as glowing and credible as the CV from a first-class honours degree graduate, has paid off. It is hard bringing up a rebel, unless you are able to sit back and watch them make their own way, which I had to do when Ben was 11. My programming wasn't his, however hard I tried.

Which personality type do you feel connected to? How could you adapt your learning and nutrition to your personality? As a questioner, perhaps you need to know why. Why are you asking me to do this? Simply because I want to discover your triggers.

Know your triggers

Who are your triggers? Is it your mum, siblings or a close friend? Do you look for approval from your children, or need it from your partner? What emotions trigger your eating habits?

- Do you have a tendency to eat the wrong things when you are bored?

- Do you turn to food when you are upset, stressed, anxious, worried, or feeling sorry for yourself?

- When are you more likely to use food as a comfort? Is it an 11am cake and coffee ritual?

- Where do you make poor choices? At home, because it is 'for the kids'?

- Do you eat 'badly' because nothing else is available or because you lack the time and inclination to prepare something nutritious?

- Are you aware of your own standard repeat comments? Take the time to write them down, journal them.

For instance, whenever I go 'home' for the weekend or see my sisters, I am suddenly my 17-year-old self again. The one who is the bossy, big sister. The situation triggers my old behaviour pattern. Or perhaps it is the meet-up with your university or college friends — do you suddenly become that beer-swigging, tequila-shooting, brash, loudmouth who loves to argue about politics? OK, maybe that one is just me. The friends trigger a consumption pattern.

The point is that circumstances and people can bring you right back to old buried emotions that can domino into destructive behaviours. Just as a distinctive smell can bring back a strong memory, situations and people can bring out certain behaviours in you. Watch for them, be aware of them and, as explained before, once you are aware of them you have the choice to change them.

Trigger awareness is enough to create new behaviour

If you know that Aunt Flo (your well-meaning but pushy aunt) makes you feel guilty and keeps insisting you eat shop-bought, plastic-tasting cake, then either avoid Aunt Flo or prepare a polite excuse before you go. Even better, look at Aunt Flo as an opportunity to test your new gorgeous self-awareness, rather than an event to be avoided. Diets often mean avoiding social situations because you can't trust yourself. You miss out eating at your family or friend get togethers. You can't live your life like that. Get used to hanging out with Aunt Flo and adapting the situation to work for you. You are in control.

Own your clean slate

It is time to move on and clean the slate, remove the guilt of the crimes for which your parents, siblings and past experiences convicted you. Feel liberated in the new version of you: past failures are learning experiences and your new adventure awaits.

Old friends can hold you stuck as well. If your best mate has struggled with her weight for decades and you move on to a healthier lifestyle, you may carry a subconscious feeling that you are abandoning her. You may feel disloyal to her and feel guilty.

Another possibility, if you do become that gorgeous girl that you were meant to be, will your shine of success be too much for others? Is there a message to your subconscious that you must dumb down your efforts or even your genius because you will make others feel or look bad? Is it safer to receive empathy and sympathy from your friends rather than jealousy? Good girls don't make mates jealous, they comfort others by being less. The good girl syndrome climbs out again: be liked, look after others and keep yourself small, don't push your happiness into other people's faces.

This new way of being is far from your good girl norm. When you avoid uncomfortable feelings, you stay stuck in your old way of thinking. In turn, the universe shows you more and more of this same pattern. If you assume that loved ones will be hurt by your successful, gorgeous figure, then the universe will bring those people to you.

It is the law of attraction playing out again. What you think about you bring about: even fat cells attract more fat cells. While it is impossible to filter every thought, I know from experience that simply asking gently, without anguish, you will receive everything you ask for. It is how I finally got my babies.

What is your excuse?

We all have an excuse pattern. An excuse for not getting up in the morning, leaving a big project to the last minute or waiting until you have reached the next level of success before relaxing.

What is your weight loss excuse?

When I first started working as a coach, I took it upon myself to solve every one of these excuses until I realised that everybody's excuse is different. I adore the way a gorgeous girl's brain works. If you want something, there are all sorts of things you'll devise to get it.

If you don't want to change your 'healthy' fruit juicing habit or telly and crisps habit, you will create a wall of comfort and personal reasoning around your choices. Eventually I gave up unpicking each one of these excuses: you are way too clever for me.

Change has to come from you. I realise that now. I simply need to show you the excuse and let you do the processing. I won't give you the solution to your wall, but I will be able to show you the excuse. I have seen and heard them all. You are really quite brilliant at excuses.

What excuse do you use daily to justify why you can't do something, like getting fitter? When you are asked to help your best friend to put together a charity event, what is your brand of excuse?

Of course, some tasks are way out of your ability or comfort level, so you can be excused the odd opt out – like running a marathon in six weeks' time. But what about those challenges or dreams you have that you can absolutely do if you set your mind to it? If you spend the time and lay out your dreams and think about what you really want from life, what is actually stopping you?

When your morning alarm goes off and you lie in bed listening to your own stream of thoughts (or in my case babble), what is your inner dialogue saying? What excuse are you using to justify why you can't get up and go for a walk in the rain? Your excuses are decaying your dreams and I am here to fight for your inner gorgeous girl that is screaming to get out.

Which excuse thread resonates?

"I don't care what anyone thinks. [12] I am very happy with the way I look. I don't want to be skinny because people love me the way I am. Anyway, if I was skinny it would be too much like hard work and I would never be able to keep it up, why should I even bother?"

Or the excuse, "Life is too difficult. My husband never supports me. If he doesn't come on board with my new regime, then I can't stick to it. The changes I want to make are beyond my control, in fact, my entire life is beyond my control."

"I was born fat. I was born this way and I can't behave any differently. My mum struggled with her weight and confidence her whole life and I am exactly the same. There is nothing I can do about it. I have the fat gene." The truth is we all have the fat gene; your lifestyle decides whether it is switched on or not.

"I can't help it. I am a victim of others' behaviour. John brings cakes into the office every Friday — it is an office tradition, it is the way we bond."

Or "Everybody in my family eats crisps and chocolates. It is the way we relax, it is the way that the family come together and spend time with each other. Spending time eating crisps on the settee is our quality family time. I can't change that, it is what my kids and husband expect. The kids want biscuits in the house and if there are biscuits in the house, I have no self-control: I eat them."

Or a slightly deeper and harder one to hear is: "I'm messed up; I have had a screwed-up childhood. My mum was never around, and my dad drank; nobody cared or looked after me and my brother, so I turned to food."

How about the excuse that you are so busy and overwhelmed that you "haven't got time to change your life?" Do you have that frustration that no one is helping you or appreciating you? Nobody is noticing how hard you have to work to make your life run smoothly? Do you mope around and complain that nobody sees how hard you work? Maybe by moaning or silently putting up with the inequality gives you opportunity to watch how people don't appreciate you, which fills your 'victim bucket' to the brim.

"I am going to break," resonates a little harder than the rest to me personally. I fully understand the principle, "If you push me any further, I will break." That feeling of overwhelmed, exhausted fatigue can rule your life. However, from my own personal experience, when you reverse your psychology and feel worthy enough to care for yourself, then you will have a clearer mind, a lighter step and the ability to do all that you want to achieve in your gorgeous, happy life.

The truth is when you understand and plan your nutrition and exercise and turn off that nagging voice you will overcome the overwhelming exhaustion and fatigue. You will have the energy to have a productive work flow and loving relationships with your loved ones. You will have the mental energy to take on that overbearing boss at work and break through the cloud of brain fog.

Once the penny drops, you will realise that the only thing holding your amazing self back is you. You are making the excuses and shutting doors. Once you understand that these comments are simply excuses, you will be free.

Lift the veil, understand that you are making excuses and move forward with love and respect for your gorgeous body. Set up realistic steps forward, not desperate, dramatic steps forward.

Be 'excuse aware'

This exercise in 'excuse awareness' is all about realising that you are doing just that. Making excuses. Making lame excuses to not live the life you have always wanted. You are holding yourself back by uttering, "I will get that promotion when I have lost 6lbs."

Making unconscious excuses means that your life is on autopilot. You can have the freedom to be who you are meant to be and who you want to be only when you first fully understand how you speak to yourself and what excuses you make.

Learn to catch your thoughts and feelings. Watch for your attitudes and points of view that are leading back to your old perceptions. Whenever a thought comes into your mind that you no longer want to hold, let it fly straight back out, as if it were a bird trapped in a birdcage. Open the door and let it fly away, with no detachment. [13]

What is your motivation madness?

The value of aligning with your personal values to create your motivation was something we learned from Linda in a previous example. Once you have understood what your underlying drive and passion is, then getting out bed in the morning will be easy: to achieve the prestige of looking and feeling great, having more energy and self-esteem.

Sarah, a fellow runner, explains that her motivation is to be fit and flexible in her old age. She wants to keep going, using her body and staying active for as long as possible.

Add in positive behaviour and work with small habits, rather than using the diet mantra of denial. Rather than looking at what you can't eat, look at what you can eat in your diet. That is much more appealing. I can enjoy peanut butter and dates, rather than focusing on never eating pizza again. Your momentum starts with small steps and builds on that to total transformation.

When striving to achieve a goal you need to know the reason behind your objective. That's because your 'why' holds the secret to your motivation and commitment.

What does good health mean to you?

Do you want to get a gold star from your doctor for your cholesterol count or get rid of your belly? Or perhaps your good health means feeling less sluggish and depressed? Do you want great skin or to slow down the signs of ageing?

What will greater vitality add to your life? Do you want to feel sexier to your spouse or new partner? Do you want the energy and stamina to be able to play with your children or grandchildren without getting tired? Do you want to lose weight to fit into that gorgeous pair of jeans? To look great on your holiday? Or to avoid the lifestyle disease that took one of your parents?

Your goals should match your values. They are not 'should' goals, as in "You should lose 6lbs." Instead you *must* want them badly enough that you are fully responsible for gaining them.

Willpower has a short span

Willpower has a lifespan: it needs recharging like a battery. Every morning your willpower cup is full to the brim. It is strongest at the beginning of the day and wanes throughout your decision-making day. Any decision-making process – whether it is what shoes to wear or whether to eat a birthday cake or filling out your tax form – will deplete your willpower cup. If your day is filled with countless little questions and requests, drop by drop your cup will be drained until it is depleted, and anything goes. You will agree to anything.

"Let's go down the pub or bar and dance on the tables," or "Of course you can have 12" pizza, Johnny, and get me two while you're there." These are all signs that your willpower cup is drained.

Plan to move out of bad habits

Before you take the last dregs from your willpower cup, set your intention, plan your way out of bad habits. Prepare for when your willpower is at its lowest by putting together a plan. Plan to avoid low points and temptations. Exercise at the beginning of the day before your brain has woken up. Kick off your feel-good endorphins by succeeding at your first task of the day: perhaps a half-hour home workout or outside in the sun, wind or rain.

Exercise in the morning and you will settle into your day with a positive frame of mind.

Willpower will also be replenished when you rest, taking a 10-minute power nap during the day, or meditating perhaps. A walk will reset, recharge and renew your willpower.

Find your success in commitment to your goals.

Successful people tend to use a carrot goal rather than a stick one. [14] Stick is a pain motivator, the route that a restrictive diet takes. It goes along these lines: "You will be fat forever if you don't stick to this painful meal plan. If you don't make a separate choice from your family, sit at a different table or eat weird, processed crap that is low fat, you will not succeed."

EXERCISE

Rearrange these words and make your own sentence:

Doom, gloom, penance, stick, failure, beat, diet.

A carrot approach involves embracing your new future, the possibility of being able to fulfil your sporting challenge, for example, a run for charity or completing the three peaks (Priscilla), or being able to walk into the room and everybody says, "Wowzers!" (Sandra). Your carrot is a journey of fulfilment and self-understanding and love and it is a path forward rather than running away from where you have been. A sustainable positive, planned change rather than coming from a place of pain.

Commitment is harnessed when you have spent time accepting yourself today, honoured who you are and made yourself aware of your triggers. Simply having a more open emotional awareness of yourself will help to acknowledge your own inner critic. [15] Recognise the chatter and aid your recovery, so that you will be able to drop your addiction to worry, criticism and blame. Life choices will be easier once you consider how you want to live in the future. Acknowledge your 'why' and your commitment to your goals and include a spiritual component towards mending your heart. [16]

Listen to your inner mentor

Look to your inner mentor for advice. Dream big and listen to that voice in your head; she may start quiet, but the more you pay attention the bigger she will grow. Listen and be guided by her. Your emotions are a guide to your intuition and that will pave your way to healthy, gorgeous success.

Be guided by Queen Flow, not Aunt Flo

Jane was always being told, "You are way too emotional." After hours of dissecting the latest catastrophe in her life

– a dissatisfied customer, a traffic incident, a playground argument or something equally major – her mum would say, "Get over it, don't be so emotional."

And yet your emotions are your inner compass; you should live by your instincts. Yet so many have subdued their emotions to 'fit in', allowing negative voices to reign because they have never been outed. Your inner mentor is who you will be in five years' time; she talks sense. She holds the key, she is a supreme being who needs to be heard. Queen Flow.

I am always interested in the 'shut the fridge' stance. I've heard it from weight loss coaches and fitness instructors where the stick approach is: "Exercise harder, put it down, it is all down to willpower." That feels as if it is missing the entire point of why you go to the fridge in the first place and it says more about them than you. Find out why you feel sad, tune in and listen to your excuses, recognise them as such, then you are free either to work towards your gorgeous vision or think, "Not today, today I need bread and jam." Some days we all need crumpets, with hot butter and jam.

Be slow, be consistent and consider the Chinese proverb, "Don't be afraid of going slowly, only be afraid of standing still."

Five frogs sit on a lily pond. One decides to jump off – how many are left? *

---

*Five. They only *decided*, they didn't take action, so let's jump off the lily pond together. [17]

CHAPTER 2

The truth is everything is going to be OK for you

Coming to terms with the fact that you are in your own way can be a painful realisation. Even if you can't immediately associate with some of the points raised in the previous chapter, perhaps they have created a small shift in your thinking. Trust your process.

This chapter is about reassurance and the theme of the book, everything is going to be OK and managing your health and weight loss is easy, once you get behind it with conviction, self-compassion and love for yourself and your gorgeous body.

Socrates apparently said, "The unexamined life is not worth living." I am a keen navel-gazer: I adore knowing why people create their own environment. It is an interesting truth knowing that your environment is created by you. Your brain manifests in your outer world what your inner world is experiencing. For instance, if you believe that the world is unfair, then you will have only the cognitive awareness that reassures you that the world is indeed unfair. You will be shown examples that increase that perception, you will watch the news and see that unfair things are being created by very bad people.

On my website, I offer one-to-one health consultations, which can be incredibly powerful sessions and can lead to further work together or simply an understanding and clarity. There is an application process and I vet these applications carefully. Recently an applicant completed my application form and filled it with negativity, complaining how unfair life was and commenting, "I have seen your website, it is unfair, lots of people can use your services, why are you limiting it?" Unfortunately I rejected this application, which resulted in another 10 insulting, negative comments. I have to look after my own Queen Flow; working with that level of negativity is hard. I understand sadness, but accusatory negativity is too much: ownership and self-development comes first.

If you offer your brain a simpler, happier version of the world, like the fictious *La La Land*, it sounds simplistic and a bit out of touch with reality, but it can become your reality. If you aim to live in an optimistic way, you will see the best qualities in people. Later on I will discuss more about the scientific basis for this, as well as the spiritual element. It works on your neurosignature – remember that? The way your brain wires together and creates a brain groove. I do love a groovy brain: I can imagine it singing and dancing along to Abba.

Be comforted, allow your thought processes to unfold

Recognising that you create associations in your life based on how you perceive the world (from the last chapter) may well represent a breakthrough for you. Or perhaps it may be something you are aware of but not something you practise yet. This chapter will elaborate on how to practise feeling your emotions and being comforted by that. It is OK to feel sad; it can be safe and acceptable. It is regularly ignoring the sadness, covering it up, that creates long-term damage.

Psychologists explain that an emotional feeling of emptiness is a common eating disorder clue. The pun is intended. That empty feeling that you fill with food, but it is not your stomach that is empty, it is your emotions. Feeling emotionally bankrupt, because you have given of yourself for so long that you can't remember how you feel about anything. Being unable to make a decision for yourself is a manifestation of this. I've got the 'give everything' badge, T-shirt and mug. My hubby pointed out to me years ago that I gave so much to my clients, there was nothing left to give at home. That was a big full stop moment for me.

Your inner child needs reassurance and the comfort of the home. We are biologically programmed to have a nature that nurtures and cares and stays close to home. *The Chimp Paradox* [1] explains that the female chimp survived by being welcoming and homely, looking after the brood and being a useful part of the community. A self-interested chimp that had a bit of confidence and exuberance was pushed out of the community. Self-confident women are out on a limb; society isn't keen on the individual female, however she shows up. It is our programming, which is OK, because when you know that, you can see that others are working from their 'chimp' rather than their higher self. *Sex in the City*, ITV's *Loose Women* and others are doing a great job of diminishing those programming issues. Again another apt pun, I am becoming better at these.

Emptiness

Recognising that your eating issues are based on your instant emotions is generally easy to detect. You are probably aware that you eat when you feel emotional or something has not gone your way. What is more interesting to dive into is why.

What was the emotion and why have you chosen to eat the big bag of crisps? Is it because you have worked hard and need a treat? Is identifying your real needs and finding a treat that would satiate those needs just resonating a little too deep and perhaps requiring more mental cognition that you want to give it? Comfort food can be immediate and feel gratifying. But what you really need is to sit down and think or cry. Perhaps all you really want is something or someone to love you? Then the crisps become part of the problem, but they are not the cause. The emotion was there first, crisps were how you decided to deal with the emotional issue.

Are you eating because Fred was really rude to you at work today and processing that hurt takes too much thought? Maybe your inner dialogue goes along these lines…

"You understand that Fred is a prat, but why he should bother you is strangely interesting. You are much too clever to worry about Fred; you are even aware that what he said wasn't true and perhaps covering up for a mistake he made. Are you eating because you are indignant and want to smash Fred's face in? Nobody deserves to be spoken to like that. Are you eating simply because you can't be bothered to think? You know there is a deep reason and he has triggered a previous incident, but hey, you are knackered, and the crisps are calling."

Eating through emotions is normal: everybody does it. In some instances, it is probably the safest route – eat rather than smash your way through life. Punching Fred's nose creates more anxiety and trouble this time with the police.

TOP TIP

Being aware of your thoughts is the first step to changing your personal psychology. You don't need to do anything other than observe and notice how you feel.

Unfold your emotions

Navel-gazing is interesting; introspection is very revealing. Push your introspection forward by being curious rather than simply ruminating. Don't take decades over the same work; ask questions, move on. Being curious may throw up stuff you thought you had dealt with a long time ago.

Past emotional baggage can be in the big suitcase in the luggage department of your brain. It brings you and me to the next question: "Do you associate with your feelings from the past or have you disassociated from them and locked them away?"

If you have locked them away, it means they are still there, they just come up every now and again when you meet a trigger like a relationship break-up or a horrible boss trigger.

Once you start 'down the road less travelled', it means looking at your own reasons and thinking about what is behind your actions. This can become way more interesting. I think you are interesting; do you think your thoughts are interesting? Disassociation means being completely unaware of your actions. For instance, you might have a feeling of protection by being overweight.

Fiona fascinated me. She used to talk about women who were skinny as being 'high-maintenance', as though skinny women were whiners and whingers who demanded a lot of attention. Her genuine fear was that she didn't want to be a burden and be high-maintenance. Once Fiona could see her thinking pattern, her programming, she was free to lead the life she loved.

You may have deep, disassociated feelings – that is, you are not aware of them or you have dissociated your feelings from your actions. Fat is safe and non-threatening and feeds your 'good girl' status when really your inner psychopath wants to play, but you are too scared to let her out. Understandably, but what if she isn't a psychopath? What if she is just excitable and a bit noisy, maybe even widely creative and adventurous? But she has been stuffed in the suitcase for so long that she feels a little psychotic now.

Disassociation may mean that you have an unconscious belief that dieting can give you a sense of control: being on a diet will help you to control the mad world that you have created. If your world is busy, non-stop, you may secretly love the chaos because it means people depend on you. You feel loved, and being on a diet will add to this mysterious adventure. You can control your diet, even though you can't control your boss with his unpredictable temper or Johnny who has failed to get out of bed on time. In a world of chaos, a diet is something you can exert your control over.

Control is a sign you need emotional sustenance

Control allows your brain to focus on small things when the larger things in life feel so out of control. If you can't afford to pay your mortgage, if your boss is unpredictable or if your business is not the success that you want, then controlling little things will help to settle and sooth the disquiet in your brain.

Do you love being a drama queen? Who doesn't? It can be fun every now and again – perhaps that is why some people love to get hopelessly drunk so they can let go, be wild and let go of their inner diva. Perhaps if she came out more often during your day you would recognise her, call her out and wonder why she appeared.

Disassociation through food 'must haves'

The disassociation that in my experience is most striking relates to the foods that you absolutely can't live without or with. I am intrigued when some people are emphatic about what they will and won't eat.

Rachel often tells me, "I won't eat that, because I can't stand the texture." Anna explains, "I can't eat peas. Peas are evil. I even look around my Sunday roast and make sure none of them are hiding under my roast potatoes: they spoil a meal."

Dig deeper, gorgeous, not just under the spuds, but under the thoughts behind those comments. Let me reassure you that if you look after yourself then a whole new pea-anxiety-free world will open up. You won't sweat those little guys: you will live like a proper princess without the prosecco and have fun. Enjoy your life flow. The peas will take care of themselves.

Are you willing to trust yourself?

If you are willing to listen and trust yourself, you will begin to associate with your thoughts. "That is interesting; I didn't know that thought was there." The leap comes when you recognise your own behaviour and love yourself as you are. Acceptance of who you are is such a liberating experience.

Treating yourself with love and understanding is imperative on your health journey. If you are running five times a week or doing repetitive gym work or even dieting three times a year, it is repetitive and destructive work that is *not* moving you on. Einstein explained that the definition of insanity was doing the same thing over again and expecting different results. If you are going to the gym three times a week and you are no stronger, fitter or slimmer, then accept it and find an alternative adventure.

Feel blessed and wear funky leggings

Honour who you are; you are blessed, and you are truly loved. Let that shine out of you. Wearing the most gorgeous pair of leggings that you can when you go the gym will help. Wearing a pair of sexy leggings or a great pair of shoes to work may seem a little impractical or showy – remember Fiona and her fear of being high-maintenance – but oh my goodness, does it make you work harder.

I have carried out the research [2] which shows that wearing the right gear improves your physical performance, and wearing the right shoes definitely improves your confidence and kick-ass ability to get that client or prove that very intricate political point. Shoes matter!

The Discipline of BLISSAPLINE

Being kind to yourself is a discipline and it is a discipline that girls are not very good at acknowledging and acting upon. Perhaps that is why wearing a great pair of shoes sounds extravagant to you. What a flimsy, heretical thought – a new pair of shoes or even worse a new pair of leggings, what extravagance.

It is part of your mind shift and feeling the part. Being disciplined about looking after yourself will change your world – more about that later – but for now know that Blissapline is an art form that needs to be cultivated and is good for your mental health and requires gorgeous shoes.

Creating a positive attitude for life will change your life. It is motivating to see someone in a good mood and perhaps occasionally a little irritating; you may want them to go away and be cheerful around someone else. I appreciate that if you are feeling low then empathy is required first, before good-natured bonhomie. If you are feeling down, you need somebody to empathise with you, get on your level, feel your pain, and then move on and up.

The issue comes when you stay in that same, stuck pattern. If the friends you know keep going over the same pain, you will become stuck in that cycle. If, however, you talk to a professional, a coach or somebody who has a positive mindset, that third-person perspective will give you release. When you air your frustration or your chimp, you can thump your proverbial chest and move on. It very much depends on who you talk to you and their positive mindset.

Own your emotions

Taking responsibility is another big shift in thinking, as we discussed in the last chapter. It is easy to default to requiring others to see your pain and stress. Teresa was busy, she explained, "I am a busy marketing manager for a blue-chip company. I don't have time to prep my meals, and I just eat what is in the fridge. Anyway, it is Phillip's turn to do the shopping this week." When I enquired whether she had discussed that with him, she said, "No, I am busy; he should know that it is his turn." We had an amusing five-minute discussion that men just don't know. They simply don't; it is not on their radar.

It is hard to see the wood from the stress especially when it is in among the trees; it is difficult to see how and when to own a problem, especially when the injustice feels and is so real.

Looking at the bigger picture and wanting to improve your life will help you to get over yourself and go shopping or order online (my advice every time) and ignoring Phillip or any other equally uninterested yet grievous offender.

My own example comes in the form of socks! I have a carefully crafted obsessive-compulsive habit with clean and tidy spaces, a habit that I hone every day. Everyone else's pain is my delight. I believe Monica from *Friends* had some very good ideas on life. A clean home means a clean mind and yes, I obviously have a lot of Protestant or Catholic messages coming home to roost. With two teenage boys and a daughter in the house, my theories are tested daily.

My introspective tendency allows me to mull over whether I am bringing out my inner goddess or my inner ranting, teenage chimp when I wait five seconds before first screaming at the offender and second deciding to put the socks in the linen bin myself. The big discussion on creating a new generation of men who can look after themselves will have to wait for another day while I put the socks away.

That is how easy it is. The socks issue is a classic example of getting out of my own way, owning the problem in that the only person it annoys is me, airing my chimp by shouting about it to nobody in particular, and creating action by putting them away. Perhaps next time there will be fewer steps for me to follow?

How you feel is up to you

Everything is up to you. How you feel in life is up to you. Having a victim mentality, as we have discussed previously, will give you more to be a victim about. Ownership of your emotions is paramount. You can't control your emotions – that is not what I am suggesting. Your emotions and your thoughts are part of the funky, gorgeous being that you are. Having an awareness of your emotions is the thought-provoking part.

As suggested at the beginning, introspection reveals a lot: own that the thoughts come from you. There are thousands of examples that you can bring up at a moment's notice to verify that the world stinks and he or she shouldn't be doing that, but socks apart, if you own that the thoughts and the emotions are yours, not theirs, then you will be cured and losing weight will be easy. Whoah, hold on a minute, that is a big jump, Adele.

Reassure your inner 'Horace or Rose'

Neuroscientists[3] look at how the brain functions and can highlight why our reactions are so immediate. Simply put, your immediate reaction and emotion to any given situation comes from the fast-thinking chimp part of your brain. This part of your brain is ancient, the oldest part of your brain. It is referred to as the limbic area.

The limbic part is on autopilot. You can't do everything from scratch every day: it would be exhausting, so around 95% of what you do comes from the autopilot in your brain. Your inner teenager resides here; she can work with you or against you, depending on how she is feeling and how she has been nurtured that day, whether she is sunbathing and relaxed or on edge and jumpy. For me, your inner teenager, inner voice, inner child, chimp, your Rose or your Horace are all interchangeable and depend on your emotions for their presence. If you are calm, then Rose will go outside and sunbathe; if you are feeling shouty and upset then Rose comes out loud and strong. If you are feeling cheated, then your inner teenager, Rose, stamps her feet. They are all the same 'ego' inner voice, which needs a secure place to be heard.

The more sophisticated part of your brain, where your inner goddess resides, is called the neocortex. This part of your brain is a little more sophisticated and wants the very best of you. She waits patiently until the teenager has exhausted her foot-stomping, wailing drama, and your goddess will come up with a new action plan, your new way forward. That is why weight loss is easy – you have a gorgeous goddess on your side who is simply waiting to be heard.

Back for a moment to the teenager: this emotional, messy haired, impulsive go-getter and 'sod the consequences' kind of girl is enormous fun. She loves getting off her head, dancing on the chairs and taking off her bra. The next morning it is the goddess that talks to her calmly when the teenager is lying in tatters on the floor, bra in hand (obviously way too dramatic: you are far too sophisticated for that kind of behaviour).

The point is your inner, wild teenager needs reassurance. She is not going to miss out, she may feel that she would adore that ice cream, chocolate-coated, caramel-biscuit-topped pizza. The goddess will explain calmly that life is not all about the instant gratification when you have a higher purpose and a bigger calling.

Your vision is directed by your inner goddess and she can't be doing with pizza. But your crazy girlfriend, Rose the Chimpetta, doesn't know that. Neurolinguistic programming (NLP) works on the premise that all behaviour is good behaviour and that is a great starting point to understanding your Rose, your Horace or your Fredamenia – whichever name you give your inner teenager. She serves a purpose of keeping you safe and small. She also offers a glimmer of an insight, if you are curious. "Why do I want the chocolate-covered pizza?" goes back full circle to feeling your emotions. Allow your goddess to assess the situation and work out the best way forward for your teenager, which allows you to move closer to your vision.

How were your teenage years?

Talking to inner teenagers can be fun: they are full of sassiness and rebellion. The secret is knowing how to work with your inner teenager. Imagine how powerful she would be if she were on your side? Imagine what she would achieve and the boundaries she would smash if she were working for you?

Reassure your inner little girl

Another way of looking at the impulsive teenager is viewing her at a much younger age, say five. That wonderful age when you are totally free of inhibition and love the world and the world loves you. It might not be five.

Life can make your inner little girl very unsure and unstable. She isn't allowed ice cream every day and she is not keen on that. She will wail and jump and shout and not understand why. If it wasn't explained at five in a way that she understands, then that feeling of not having what she really wanted stays with you. The emotion stays with you, not the practical rationale, the emotion.

Kids can't compute rational thoughts, it is not the rational thought that stays with a kid. It is the emotion. Here is a clear, heartbreaking example. T was a very naughty little boy in my school when I was five. He used to follow the girls into the toilet. He had issues. The girls knew something wasn't right, but not really sure what, we didn't talk about it. We couldn't rationalise it, and to be honest it was amusing that he was so interested in us. Cheryl, my BFF, and I used to giggle. At five, it was harmless, so we thought.

While in the library one day, with the aforementioned boy, he asked us to lift our jumpers a little and show him our belly buttons, we played along. A teacher saw the incident from the internal window.

She was horrified, angry and indignant. She told the little boy off, then shouted at the girls. We cried and never forgot 'the incident' of shame. What didn't we forget? Why are the five-year-old class photos never on display? Because of the way the teacher made us feel about ourselves. We were dirty. Kids can't rationalise; they understand only the emotions they are left with. Cheryl and I were left feeling that we had done something very wrong, that we had let ourselves down. We couldn't unpick the incident and realise that the teacher could see the 'potential' of the situation or the background. We only felt the shame and internalised that pain.

Cake eating and feeling as though you are missing out is similar, if you have been told that you can't have the cake – you are fat! Or you can't have the cake because you have had enough but you really want the cake. You are always left with the feeling of wanting or the dishonour of being told you are fat.

Reassure your inner child she is OK, sometimes grown-ups are crazy and cranky and they are knackered most of the time, stressed and not rational. You are very welcome to eat cake, gorgeous girl; enjoy every last mouthful. You can eat cake whenever you want. As long as it is home-made, and you have had a snack of protein and fat before hand – sorry, got twitchy. You are of course allowed cake, if it makes you feel groovy and it is home-made.

And yet cake will easily dissolve into insignificance when you have your eyes on a bigger slice of life's cake, when you know what you are here to do. The difference is when you are told that you can't, you waste time arguing that battle rather than being open to your big life dream.

Deepak Chopra believes that "everyone has a purpose in life, a unique gift to give to others." What is yours? Is it to be the best entrepreneur or business owner of all times – hallelujah yes! To have a well-respected career? Is it to be a mother? I struggled with that one for 10 years! Or is it to guide and heal the world in some way? Profound or insular and personal to you, it doesn't matter, gorgeous one, as long as you know what it is and hold it to your heart.

What is your life quest?

What makes you so mad you want to release your inner teenager and smack Fred in the chops again? Poor Fred. Acting with purpose, loosens the shackles of your procrastination. Passion is purpose and purpose has determination. Determination and focus are your power tools. I have worked with hundreds of women and my one goal is not weight loss – it is finding their key. What drives you?

For example, gorgeous, beautiful Jemima is a fully qualified architect. She qualified and yet she became very stressed and disillusioned with the company she was working with and decided to leave it all behind and fell in love and happily pregnant. She had a beautiful daughter and married a very handsome, clever lawyer, moved to a different country and had a wonderful life. Clever plan.

Not quite. She contacted me when her daughter was a screenager and had an active, busy running schedule. Her daughter was involved, at a high level, in the country's athletic events. Running had also been Jemima's childhood passion. She helped and promoted her daughter's passion because she knew and understood the joy that the sport had given her. The problem was that she wasn't the active mum role model she wanted to be for her daughter. She had lost herself. She had lost her self-confidence and her figure and of course her old vitality and energy.

Diving deep, we worked out that it wasn't the being at home mum that bothered her: it was the fact that she hadn't dealt with the stress and the bruising that her confidence had taken when she'd walked away from her role as a professional woman. With her daughter living her dreams, what were Jemima's dreams? She wondered if she had done the right thing.

Of course, nobody would doubt that bringing up her wonderful daughter was the right path for her, but now she needed to reclaim her self-worth and self-love. The gorgeous habits were easy peasy for Jem and she loved the motivation of working with the group. She had forgotten what a wonderful asset her ambitious drive was, and that her resilience was formidable. She knew what to eat, of course; that was easy. Jem had simply needed the passion. She found it in coaching. Jem has rekindled her love of running and has become an athletics coach, organising trips and speakers for her daughter's athletics club. She runs and loves life. She has rekindled her excitement and her old devotion to herself and her running.

Maslow's hierarchy of needs – secondary school geography – remember?

I remember learning this in geography at school, the higher actualisation at the top and shelter and food at the bottom of the triangle. The model is based on fulfilling your basic needs of food and comfort and then you climb the hierarchy, and once you have everything then you will realise what life is about and reach self-actualisation. This model of thinking is based on scarcity. Everything will fall into place once you have climbed the ladder and reached the top. It is a model of fighting and climbing your way to the top, with limited resources. [4]

This scarcity model pushes you into believing that you won't get what you want until you have climbed the ladder and then you will rock. Instead invert the triangle and come from a different place. Rock right now. Self-actualisation is happening in India right now. They love life, smile and wish you love and wellbeing in a simple morning hello – namaste. They have self-actualisation and we have the food!

Coming from a place of lack and attack is not worthy of your inner goddess; she is so much more sophisticated in her high heels and new Lycra leggings. She is a class act. She has her head in the sky and feeling and living her vision. Her sense of purpose allows her to think beyond achieving the basics.

My version of the hierarchy of needs is much simpler. Your health comes from your mindset first, and your physical activity and your nutrition will fall into place once your inner goddess is in charge.

Adele's Get Gorgeous works from the inside out.

Starts with your mindset and self-acceptance, then with support your nutrition and finding exercise you enjoy falls simply into place.

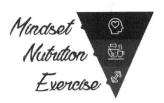

Credit: Almond Fabros via Upwork

Living in India for 16 days made me a deep thinker and a careful appreciator of all things spiritual and of India. Well, come on, 16 days would. I adored the love and kindness, the smiles, the colour and the humility. I also fell in love with the sense of industry: I felt that everyone was an entrepreneur. No need to feel guilty about working hard in India, everyone is, but with grace and kindness and a sense of purpose to their higher good. It is infectious.

One picture that stays in my head forever involved the dangerous world of the tuk-tuk. They are exhilarating, fun and wonderful. There are crashes and near-death experiences every day, but what I found fascinating is that nobody is driving at the speeds we see on our roads.

A granny will walk colourfully into the middle of a roundabout, along with a slow-moving cow, a hog, three buses of kids and a couple of heavily decorated trucks, and the granny has the attitude, "You hit me and you will have very bad karma – get out my space." She knows her worth; drivers move round her, as do the dogs, the hog, the sacred cows and the articulated lorries.

The chap who whizzes past on his motorbike with his girlfriend has immaculately groomed hair, looks like a film star and knows it. He waves at the middle-aged, gawping women, and throws us a smile. His girlfriend laughs at his nonchalance and pats his beautifully coiffured hair. He knows his worth and she is happy with hers.

A recent newspaper article summed up purpose and self-worth beautifully – a young writer on the BBC website wrote about her experiences of dieting. She had done them all, including the Body Coach, and she had lost and regained weight and failed and started again. Then she noticed. She got involved in a project, something that really ignited her interest, she was lost and enthralled and guess what? Her weight fell off. [5]

Dieting creates a negative cycle that damages your self-esteem. Dieting is short term, instead of changing the way you eat forever to give you the results you crave. Change takes time and perseverance, but when you align your changing behaviour with a higher purpose, guided by your intuition, when you trust yourself, change is easy.

Repetitive diets rob your self-esteem

Repetitive dieting does not work. Repeating the same cycle of loss and gain hurts your confidence. Can I ask you gently to move on, draw a line in the sand and learn from your mistakes? Eat differently, eat intuitively, listen to your body and understand what gives your body strength and power. Trusting yourself rather than others may make you feel insecure and push you to the edge of your comfort zone. When you go to the edge of your comfort zone, you encounter fear. Diets can be a crutch, a small comfort in your world of fear.

And yet the biggest resistance comes from the way you eat. Most of us don't want to change: we want results, but without the big lifestyle overhaul. I am often asked for a little adaptation here or there – what milk in my tea? What are your tips for fibromyalgia or what two little things can I change about my diet? When I talk about macros and intuitive eating, I meet resistance and fear. Most people can't believe that weight loss can be that simple; they almost want a complicated answer.

Following the same behaviour is much easier than making a change. Even a small change in routine can be difficult. There is comfort in the same eating patterns, or diet patterns. Perhaps on a deeper level there is also a comfort of some sort in eating differently from the other members of the family.

Perhaps there is a disassociated, unexplored and invested interest in weighing pasta. There is comfort in eating apart from the rest of the family – I am a good girl, look at me following the rules, I work so hard, I have this 'weight' affliction, notice me. Where is that voice coming from, your goddess or your little girl who has been told she is not allowed biscuits?

Radical change is not required, simply adding new habits and behavioural tweaks, then watching the better habits compound and create a transformation. Past diet failures are a clue to your personal healing; don't step back into the flawed diet plan that is no longer serving you. Reflect and make a longer lasting change; incorporate small positive habits.

Act as if it is impossible to fail

Look at the times in your life where you have succeeded [6]. The great promotion at work, the job that fell into your lap, the book writing that came easily, the client that loved you and wrote a glowing report. Look at when you were mega successful and appreciated for it.

Look for the bright spots. I remember clearly the story in *Switch* [7] because it resonated and had a profound effect on me at the time of reading it, because it described the action and behaviour that I was using. My methodology was a little bit different from the norm. I stood out and I wasn't comfortable.

The original research was based in 1950s Vietnam. After the war, malnourishment was rife, the kids were starving, and the country looked doomed and on the brink of a crisis. Among the starvation statistics, there were a few measurements that stood out as 'bright spots', where the kids were not starving but thriving.

The researchers looked deeper and interviewed the parents. They discovered that the Vietnamese meal culture was based on family meals, three times a day. This structure was based on the requirements of the adults, as they were bringing in the food and providing security for the family.

However, a few families did things differently. These 'bright spots' allowed the kids to eat when they wanted, because the children were malnourished and therefore unable to eat a huge meal with the family. They needed encouragement. The parents of these kids fed them. They spoon-fed their kids nutritious food. They allowed the child to decide when they were hungry and intuitively followed their instinct.

These kids thrived. In the bigger picture of the western world, following the kids' intuition may not be good advice, they would eat candy floss and cake. But the message of feeding your child, literally spoon-feeding nutritious food, is a message I took to heart.

I encouraged my kids to eat spinach when other mums gave up. "What muck are you serving?" I felt challenged by refusing to give my kids 'orange-coloured kid food'. If Ben struggled with his fish or cabbage, I sat patiently with him and waited.

The 'bright spot' story resonated for another reason. Fattening the child meant little and often, grazing. The fattening and little often evidence struck me as curious. This is contrary to the current thinking, but it sparked a grain of truth – your body needs time to rest and digest.

Look at the times when you thrived, what was different about that time? Did you feel passionate about the cause you were involved with? That is your bright spot. Be aware when your health shone through.

Success has a framework

Stepping into your dream, allowing your inner goddess to set your overriding vision will steady you through periods of fear and uncertainty. Vision – your big why, what is your reason for obtaining your goal? Then make sure your vision matches your values. If you think a paleo diet is a good idea but you are a vegetarian, that is not going to work for you.

Chunk down your vision into goals and create new habits around your goals, such as exercising every Monday at 2pm. Look at your past successes. When have you been successful and how can you adapt that success to work now on this problem?

Admire who you are right now and look at the resources that you have so you can play to your personal strengths. Are you a great team player? Then choose a sport or an activity that depends on your being part of a team. If you are frustrated waiting for others to decide what time they are going running, set your alarm and write in your diary when *you* are going to run and motivate yourself.

Meet your thoughts with love and kindness and know that they will offer you a path and your actions will unfold. Investigate with interest and humour and be flexible. So, it didn't go as you planned today – no sweat, you can be on target in the future.

Flexible thinking is a skill you can learn to love and will help you to heal. Reward yourself; sometimes that reward will be cake and other times simply giving yourself love and reassurance. You may even respond better to a 'well done' loop back. Reassurance rather than cake – did that go well, great job, let's do it again tomorrow.

If it is important and imperative to you that you value honesty, then be honest with yourself and look at when you are manufacturing your truth or exaggerating to yourself. Acting with integrity and being 100% comfortable with who you are, living by your word, will change how you see yourself and upscale your self-confidence.

Small changes have a profound effect

A rolling ball gathers momentum, but Newton says it better: "An object in motion stays in motion, whilst an object in rest stays at rest." Get started with small habits. They may feel inconsequential, but over time a little trickle can erode rock. "Elephants don't bite, mosquitos do," which is how *The Compound Effect* [8] describes it. A habit plus consistency plus time will make a radical difference to your life.

Small poor choices left unattended will lead to long-term consequence. For example, Fiona, Debra and Sam have very different long-term consequences because of short-term actions. Fiona introduces some positive habits into her life, she starts to drink more water, consume more protein, becomes aware that fat needs to be included in her diet. She drops a few carbs like hot potatoes and begins to improve her level of activity.

Debra, on the other hand, is quite happy as a plodder; she is doing OK and doesn't need to change anything. Life is satisfactory.

Sam loves a drink, and adds an extra glass of wine on a Friday night. She loves it and she deserves it – she works hard. She can't really be bothered with exercise; she is OK managing her weight with food. She knows when she has had enough and goes on a quick diet every few months to get rid of the extra weight. Sam loves a Netflix series, she has bought a massive telly to help her enjoy the latest one.

Five months later and there is no discernible difference: Sam, Debra and Fiona are on the same trajectory. Ten months later small changes begin to appear. Two years later, Sam has gained a lot of weight and is two stone heavier than she was a couple of years ago. She has bad skin and her memory feels ropey. Her energy is at an all-time low and the diet she puts herself on every now and again isn't working any more. Her kids are addicted to the big telly and they are watching the latest Netflix series. Sam feels that life is a bit too difficult. Where is the wine?

Debra has changed nothing, life looks the same – no successes and just life as it always was.

Two years later, Fiona feels great. She has a successful business, she is aware that her mood is good, and her family have their ups and downs, but with a clear head they get through things. She has lost weight. She does something active every day, like walking to work, and uses the stairs. She feels fairly fit. She feels younger than she did two years ago and is convinced she looks it as well. The future looks good.

Small, incremental changes to your habits will change the course of your life.

The truth is everything is going to be OK with you. Reassure your inner child and your teenager; talk to your goddess, who has a plan (and it may involve very expensive leggings).

CHAPTER 3

Happiness starts
from right now

Neuroscience, the study of how the brain works, tells us that 'cells that fire together wire together', which means if you are in a positive frame of mind most of the time, your little arms in your brain cells (dendrites) will poke out from the cells and connect with other brain cells and you will fire off more happy cells.

If you are feeling grumpy, dissatisfied, that your doctor didn't look after you, that the world is a dangerous place, a 'victim mentality', your dendrites shrink back, connections are not made with any new cells and new ideas won't form. You stick with a fixed mindset. The world is crap, I'm crap, nothing will ever change.

Forced positivity is hugely annoying. We all know that, but your brain processing doesn't. Simple happiness tools, such as kindness, can make a huge impact on your life. Little acts of kindness that sometimes nobody knows about can make you feel fantastic: giving away a car parking ticket, paying for a coffee for the person next to you in the queue, giving someone a compliment, smiling at a stranger or offering the delivery chap a warm cup of tea or coffee. The kindness you offer to others will open up your whole day and shift your mental thinking. Being happy will allow you to achieve anything, with an "I can do this!" attitude.

According to Maya Angelou, "People don't remember what you said, people don't remember what you did but they remember how you made them feel." Did you make that shopkeeper feel happy and the waiter smile, or did you get peed off at the supermarket checkout? It happens. Simply think about investing in yourself and little random acts of kindness by you will fill up your happiness bank.

Scientists [1] report that you have an increase in the happy hormone serotonin when you show kindness to another. Both of you receive that boost to your happy hormone.

Avoiding confrontation is important to your mental health and throughout this chapter I will show how to do this for your physical health as well.

Setting up to be happy

Living by your word and your own integrity will set up some positivity ground rules, which in turn will help with your own self-esteem and happiness.

Truly listening to the person you are chatting with will help ground you and create more meaningful communication. If they are coming from a place of upset, hear their pain and just watch your teenager. If you are unable to listen quietly and your inner teenager is jumping up and down angrily because of something that is being said, you have found a personal trigger.

Oh, how exciting, this is a trigger, an insight, a deeper understanding of you. Of course, in the heat of the moment it is hard to stop and listen to the trigger, but perhaps afterwards when you recall the argument, you'll notice the trigger within you.

In time you will avoid the triggers and be able to listen to the person, their point of view. It may be hard at first but avoid making the assumption that you are right, and they have got the world all wrong. I know you are right, you are a goddess but just give the other person five minutes to air their chimp, their grievances. If it is too difficult, be selfish and walk away.

Be clear in what you want and need. If you feel that a conversation will be antagonistic, spend a few moments considering what you are going to say. This comes under a habit interruption strategy – ping on the arm with an elastic band, or a simple phrase, "I love myself", will give you a moment to stop and reflect and come from a place where your higher self resides.

Be courageous and speak your mind, which is difficult for most women. Courage usually comes in a spurt of anger because we are so unused to speaking our opinion and feeling heard. Be courageous and kind with yourself. Ask for what you need. [2]

Susan lost her husband five years ago. They had been devoted to each other and she had nursed him through his painful illness and last few years. Before he became ill, if he was first home at night he did all the cooking, before she arrived back from work. They were compatible; he was dependable and the love of Susan's life. When he died, she described herself as lost. When she first approached me, she burst into tears: she was still grieving, but said, "How ridiculous is that! It's five years on."

Later, when we had worked together for a while and she had lost two stone in weight, Susan reflected back on this conversation and explained that nobody wanted to hear her pain. "Nobody wants to see you upset, it isn't unkindness, I don't like seeing anyone upset." She acknowledged that her grief was blocking her life and was even questioning her reasons "for being around". This was very delicate, and I wanted to know more.

Susan explained she had been in a bad place, but the gorgeous process had given her small wins. She felt she had a focus and understood food. These accomplishments made her appreciate that she could do this, she could move on. A simple success, an easy win, made all the difference and changed the direction of her entire life. She adores and talks to her beloved often. We talked about respecting and loving him from a place of love. He wanted her to be happy, rather than live in a place of pain.

Be courageous and ask questions. If you are not sure about how somebody is feeling or how you have interpreted them, be curious.

Be happy right now

Happiness right now will make you more productive. Happiness in the now, being comfortable with who you are, will make you more motivated. Happiness will see you become more efficient and effective in your actions.

The positive psychology movement in the 1960s described that pleasurable engagement in a process will help you to progress [3].

If you are happy with the food you are eating, if you are happy that your vision is in place and you want to get there, then you will be more productive, inventive and clever about how to achieve this. This theory isn't just based in psychology; it is based on neuroscience as well. Let's talk about the interesting psychology bit first, how positive, optimistic people are more likely to excel in life.

Nuns living in the Notre Dame Cathedral in the 1970s were questioned on entering the convent. Their frame of mind was assessed, through a number of sophisticated psychological tests to determine whether the nun had a positive or negative outlook on life, such as, "Are you generally a happy person or unhappy person?" The testing was rigorous. Then 20 years later, they looked at the nuns' life expectancy. Hazard a guess at the results. The happier nuns lived longer. [4]

In another example, doctors diagnosed patients' illnesses more effectively when the doctors were given a small treat before meeting and diagnosing a patient's symptoms. A simple happiness boost in the form of a lollipop was all that was required. In the control group, doctors were given no lollies. The happy, lolly doctors were 34% more likely to come up with the correct diagnosis compared to the no happiness boost lolly doctors. The moral of the story is: smile at your doctor, compliment her or him on their new shoes. [5]

What was interesting about this research was the discovery that the happiness boost was really small. It didn't have to be a big incentive. Small happiness boosts could be looking forward to your favourite film, an act of kindness, exercise, creating a new experience, or even doing something that is your signature strength. What are you good at? Motivating people, looking after people, great with the community, maths? Doing a small task that exhibits your signature strength will give you a happiness boost.

EXERCISE

Write down five things that you like about yourself.

What is your signature strength?

Sales performers are the same: an optimistic salesperson is more likely to be effective if they start the day with a smile. Why not give enforced happiness a go? Having a positive mindset is vital when you are being guided to exercise and create a new eating habit. Get behind your goals, make them your goals and have an invested interest in achieving them.

Why you need to celebrate your success

Happiness gets you started and will motivate you into action. Your mindset will help you carry your actions through and defines your reality. With around 20,000 pieces of information thrown at you each day, your brain acts as a spam filter.

Watch the news and you will be demoralised instantly. Listen to your friends moaning about a bad boss or a bad-tempered client and you will be upset for the rest of the day, or even the week. Lawyers and tax specialists are reputed to have the most depressing careers. Constant vigilance and looking over data to find the inconsistencies means that they are set to look for negativity. Looking for the flaws, the holes in the argument, requires a negative mindset, being stuck in a pattern of negative focus. [6]

Stay focused on your bigger vision

Business coaches often use the 'gorilla and basketball game' as an example of looking at the detail and missing the bigger picture. The consultant asks the trainees to watch a video with a blue and a red team playing basketball. At the end of the sequence, the viewers are asked how many ball passes are made by each team? At the end of the film clip after the answers are discussed, the smug consultant asks, "How many of you saw the gorilla?" Gorilla? Watching the sequence again, the trainees finally see a gorilla (man dressed as one) walking on in the background. Don't let the smug consultant get you on that one. The trainees are so busy concentrating on the passes they miss the gorilla. [7]

Similarly, I was asked to undertake some psychometric tests for a high-flying job when I was 28. The interviewer asked me to complete the questionnaire, which contained quite involved, detailed questions. I love to please and revelled in this opportunity to use my new, shiny pen. As I worked through the questions, the interviewer asked me constant questions – interruption, interruption, interruption. I became frustrated trying to do two jobs well, so I gave up, put my pen down with a decisive thump, looked at the interviewer and gave her my full attention.

She offered me the job. Who knew that was coming? I didn't take the job, by the way. I had a young son at home and the salary was too high and I was scared about not being able to look after my boy – that is another story and you can psychoanalyse my part in that.

Your mindset affects what you see in life

The unexpected events of daily life will push and move you off your target, but if your vision is clear and well-directed you will regain your ambition for success.

Another example that I absolutely adore is that of the optimist and the pessimist reading a newspaper. Research carried out on a group of people attributed two classifications: those who felt that they were unlucky in life and those who felt optimistic about life.

The two groups were asked to look through a newspaper and count up how many adverts there were in the entire paper. Their accuracy and their responses were timed. The optimists found the answer in approximately 2.3 seconds. The 'unlucky in life' participants took longer, 5 minutes. The twist in the story was that on page 2 there was a message. There are 43 adverts in this newspaper. The optimists saw the notice and the 'unlucky in life' readers missed it. The optimists also went on to earn £20 by asking the researcher for payment. Another notice at the end of the paper had alerted them that there was a reward of £20 if the reader simply asked the researcher for the cash. Again the pessimists missed it because they weren't looking; they missed the opportunities. [8]

Be curious and be open-minded and keep your wits about you, especially when asked to do a psychometric test. It is never what you think. Your brain is a spam filter. It needs to be, as there are millions of messages being directed at you every day. If you want to stay focused, limit your negative messaging and be open to positivity, which will allow new opportunities to present themselves to you.

Your mindset creates your success

If we agree that your mindset is your decision bias and can affect what you notice in life, including the opportunities, it follows that you can approach your health and lifestyle in a similar way.

Diet-orientated or purpose-orientated?

Diet-orientated means that your focus is on self-regulation, scarcity thinking, deprivation, avoidance. Diets are restrictive.

Focus on your bigger 'why', your vision, your end result (and I am not talking about a bikini shot of a model on your fridge – that has all sorts of negative connotations). I am talking about great goals, your vision for your future – travelling to New Zealand, taking your business overseas, or visiting family in New Guinea. My big personal goal for giving up booze and being fit was visiting my little sister, who lives in New Zealand and is 10 years younger. Trips to volcanos and 14-mile hikes were part of a hair-raising itinerary for me to follow. It was the impetus I needed to address my 'three glasses of wine Friday, Saturday and sometimes Sunday and maybe occasionally Thursday and a bit on Monday if I had a bad day' habit.

Purpose-meaning, orientated focus will be a bigger driving force for you. Sticking to a meal plan that has been handed to you is going to get your inner teenager riled: she will kick off. Harness your inner teenager and get her on your side.

If you are a dieter, following a meal plan, used to adhering strictly to those choices and I then offer you a reduced carb strategy, your mindset will echo, "I'll be hungry." How do you know that to be true? Is it simply because your mindset has told you?

Your inner teenager will not climb on board with a meal plan. She will hate being told what to eat and when. More importantly your inner teenager will come up with lots of self-sabotaging behaviour that you didn't see coming. She wants her own way and she will be a devious devil to get her own way. Of course, the crisps are for the kids, she tells you. Of course, that one glass of wine won't affect your vision to climb Kilimanjaro in six months' time. Of course you can do want you want, nobody can tell you what to do you. You are the queen of this moment, you feel in control in the moment, you know it won't affect you in the long run, but compound effect lets you know that you are actually stuck.

Your Inner teenager wants marshmallows

Scientists offered a hungry bunch of kids marshmallows and explained that they could eat one now or wait 10 minutes and have two. Deferred choice. What would you do? Think upon it for a moment: how about if I replace marshmallow with red wine or crisps or chocolate? Would you defer the pleasure? [9]

Results showed that the deferred gratitude group went on to greater success in life. Does that motivate you? Would you still rather have the crisps? Your inner teenager is extremely clever: respect! And that is the point. She needs to be treated with respect, not dumbing down or shouting at. Does that work with your real screenagers? Shouting at them?

Your inner teenager needs to be aired, she needs to be voiced, she needs to be heard. Give your inner teenager a little time. Recognise that you can't listen to your higher self without the inner teenager being heard first. Then you can out negotiate and outmanoeuvre her.

If you want to be stronger and influence your inner teenager, guide her from a place of growth and abundance. Show her the goodies in the distance. For example, your diet may be a feeling of hard work. You may feel as if you have a deadline to meet. Judy had her best friend's wedding coming up. She didn't want to look like the dumpy bridesmaid; she wanted to look like a healthy, happy, vibrant bridesmaid. She had been married for 15 years and wanted to show her best friend how married life had allowed her to shine. Her vision was in the future, but it felt like a lifeline to her, not a deadline. She wanted to reach her goal as a shining example of married life, looking great and radiating happiness.

Your attitude to your long-term vision will help your mindset and allow you to come from a place of love and personal understanding. Working towards your long-term health rather than the short-term immediacy of a cream cake is a lifeline.

Your mindset shapes your reality

In a very famous experiment called the 'maid effect', two groups of hotel maids were interviewed. The researchers analysed the maids' daily routine, observing their actions over a measured period. They reported back to one group of maids, "You have been incredibly active over the last two weeks, you are very fit." The second group of maids were told nothing.

A month later, the researchers returned and carried out various fitness tests and weighed the maids. They discovered that the maids in the first group had lost weight and increased their fitness levels, simply because they already believed themselves to be fit. The second group had made no improvements. [10]

Social investment is an important part your success

Your mindset and attitude are important and will encourage you on your journey. It isn't always easy to 'fake it until you make it', or 'be it until you believe it'. Yet if you surround yourself with a like-minded group of friends, it will help.

Be it until you believe it. You are, after all, the sum of the five people you hang out with. If you are in a social group with dieters who are always catastrophising about this week's weight gain or loss or complaining about the world and how awful life has turned out for them, then guess what your belief system will be? If, on the other hand, you hang out with successful, optimistic and happier friends who have a welcoming disposition, your attitude will change accordingly. Broadening your base of friends is so much easier now, with Facebook groups and online forums. Like-minded people will help you to grow and reach your true potential and fulfil your passion.

Working with a coach is another path: a third party, connected and invested in your success without your emotional drama, can take a third-person stance. This option can be very helpful to see your way through the emotional debris of your day. Your blessed friends are generally absorbed in their own vision and have a vested interest in keeping you as a dear friend, so they may not always tell you the truth or feel sufficiently distant to see what you are processing or new ideas that you are formulating.

Being a good learner

Falling up is the concept that failure is inevitable, but often leads to greater opportunities. Research shows that individuals who have survived through adversity and grow through the experience are more likely to be successful in other adventures. [11]

You know the 'stuff and nonsense' type: those people who can take on the world and come through still smiling or at least putting a brave face on a bad situation. Wallowing in a situation is required for a while, airing your grievances, expressing your deepest anxiety and releasing that negative energy into the cosmos is very important and needs to be fully expressed. You can then take the attitude that what does not kill you heals you and helps you to grow.

Falling up has shown those that face adversity and fall up have a purpose mindset and hold a strong vision for their future. Taking this concept into your everyday life, you can use the 80/20 rule or 90/10 rule whereby you allow yourself to fail or go out for the evening and splurge, enjoy yourself and feel that it is OK, you are still on the right path. This is essential for your self-esteem and for holding your course through adversity.

Diets have the exact opposite effect. You become frustrated with the restrictive lifestyle, the enforced regime. Your inner teenager gets wind of the fact that she isn't allowed to do XYZ and eventually she will rebel and demand to eat ice cream and go out and hang from the proverbial chandelier.

Working with her and bringing her along and accepting that of course life doesn't always go to plan and there will be times when you want to run amok – go for it and do it with good grace. Go into a situation with your eyes wide open, make the choice to eat cake. Use a quick habit interruption strategy: "Will this nourish me, or will this punish me?"

If the cake is with pals, home-made, looks amazing and you feel in the mood, then that cake is rewarding – enjoy. If the cake or glass of wine is happening because it's Friday night, you are exhausted, and you haven't had a good day, then wine, cake and crisps may help extinguish from memory the toerag who upset you. But guess who is actually being punished?

It is like drinking from a poison chalice and expecting the toerag to die. Let it go, reason with your teenager, take a moment, a bath if you can extend it. If you still feel like the cake or wine or whichever emotional sedative you choose, think it is what you need and you have considered your options, then go ahead with a clear conscience. Be prepared to accept that 10% or 20% of the time you need to let go.

Be a good learner

Being a good learner is all about putting yourself first, realising that you are part grown-up, part teenager and part goddess and not every day is going to go according to plan.

Being beautiful and kind to yourself when you are a good learner means that you will notice opportunities to change. You will be aware of your thinking; you will see the positive and notice the calm. A non-judgmental approach will mean that if you decide to go hell for leather then you have made the choice and you are happy with the outcomes. You'll explain that in detail to your inner goddess in the morning.

I stopped drinking about five years ago. One of the reasons, as well as imminent trip to see hyper younger sister, was my hubby leaving me dancing wildly in a pub one night – arms in the air, wild dancing on my own. No dirty dancing (I don't think) but enough for me to feel awkward the next day. Embarrassment, shame – all the emotions that Brené Brown asks us to embrace, acknowledge and drop. I became fed up of feeling the shame. There was no big misdemeanour; I simply didn't want to feel like that anymore.

Jason Vale's book opened my eyes to the fact that alcohol is very addictive, a drug. My mindset had allowed me to consider alcohol part and parcel of having fun. Looking at a wonderful view with a cold glass of wine is conditioning, social conditioning. You can admire an amazing view and feel great without the glass of wine. I love the way Jason's book is written: he talks in a very soothing, subliminal way, repeating emotions and comments. I felt as though

I were listening to a Paul McKenna hypnosis tape. He is deliberately slow and rhythmical in his writing, and for me his message went deep into my subconscious and I don't drink... very much at all and very rarely dance on tables very much at all now either. [12]

OK, on occasions I do. If I feel safe, happy and fully rested. If I know that I can cope with a three-day hangover – yes, because even two glasses of good red wine with plenty of resveratrol will make me feel glazed for a few days. If I have a clear diary. I love the taste of red wine, so very occasionally I make a conscious decision to have a couple of glasses. I enjoy it, I savour it and am happy to follow the 90/10 or 80/20 rule. Good for 90-80% of the time, hang off chandeliers for 20% of the time. Good balance.

I am happy that my long-term vision is in place and I am also happy to bend my personal rules. I do appreciate that my rules are not yours, my sentiments about alcohol are not yours. But do read Jason's book and let me know what you think.

Flexible thinking is the key to your success

Through this book and chapter, I have been asking you to rethink your mindset, your values and what you believe or feel you know to be true. Flexible thinking is a state that your brain will cultivate and is referred to as neuroplasticity – this thinking wasn't written about until 2004. The old scientific concept that you couldn't teach an old dog new tricks was universally believed, until research into brain activity presented scientists with evidence of neuroplasticity. Brain cells can adapt and reform and grow. You can learn new tricks and ways of thinking. [13]

Flexible thinking and the ability to learn represent a fundamental shift in thinking for the world of neuroscience. You can opt for another choice, rewire your brain and think in a different way if you are willing to step into the unknown and become a happy learner.

The example that comes to mind is the BBC television series with Alan Sugar, *The Apprentice*, in 2015. The contestants were down to the last two. The last challenge was to present an event with the help of the other candidates who had been eliminated in the selection process.

The two contestants were very different in their outlook and background. The young lady was university educated and looked incredibly prim − I was rooting for her. She looked like a straight-to-the point, no-nonsense, fabulous, cultivated young lady who knew her mind. She was a high-level-strategic-thinking, blue-chip, corporate girl − Vana Koutsomitis. She was the girl I wanted to be at 25. I remember the impression she made, but not much else. In my mind she was a sure-fire winner.

I remembered the other contestant very well, because he wasn't the boardroom type. Joseph Valente ran a plumbing business and was a bit of a maverick, savvy, with a lot of street sense, a bit of cheek, personable and not pushy. I think the audience loved him, in the way the British love an underdog.

The final challenge went pear-shaped. At the last moment, one of the advisers explained that the contestants needed to change their strategy. The event was already well down the road in terms of planning: most of the artwork and boards were at the printers, and food was being prepared. Yet this new information changed the entire strategy. Vana kept to her word whilst Joseph wavered; she motored on and changed nothing. Wow! I was impressed with her level-headed, direct approach. Joseph wavered and weakened in light of this new information and changed his whole strategy. Bad move, I thought; too late in the game, I reasoned.

He jolly well went on to win! Alan Sugar was impressed with his flexible thinking under pressure. As was I. He blew me away. I am not sure I would have been able to change direction at that late stage, but Joseph did. He was the hero of the hour. His presentation may not have been perfect, but his thinking was based on the latest research and information. He knew where he wanted to go, and he followed his vision, acted on new information and followed his thread and flow. He wasn't stuck.

Feel into your future dream

Your vision should follow your passion. Shining at your friend's wedding or delivering a business strategy that allows you to tell the world how your product or service will rock their world. What is your vision; what will changing your life give you? If changing the way you think and your eating habits fell naturally into place. If you were waking up at 6am every morning and jumping out of bed to exercise outside in the glorious wind, rain, sun and sleet and felt hugely alive, what would you be getting up to do?

What is your passion? Why is it important for the world to see your brilliance? Feel the emotion that your vision elicits. How does it sit with you? Excitement or nervcitement? Joyous or scared, calm your inner teenager and reach into your dream. Feel, taste, smell, hear and see it in your mind's eye. Future dreaming or future thinking means bringing your future into your now: your brain will not know the difference.

You know what I mean. When you watch a film or read a great book, you carry it with you. Your brain doesn't know that you don't actually know Jennifer Anniston: if you saw her on the street you would want to talk about Ross and how they were getting on. Or perhaps a famous New York author like Gretchen Rubin is your BFF? The point is that you feel you know that person, you feel as though you have lived an event because you have imagined it so beautifully in your mind's eye. Remember how disappointing it is to read a book and then see the film?

Visualise your future as if it were happening now – future dreaming

What will being healthy mean to you? Perhaps you want to feel that you are sexy, feel that you still have the allure? You want your hubby or partner to think you rock. Is that your motivation? Do you want stamina or energy so you can run for a bus, taxi or keep up with your kids?

Annemarie worked with me because she was the designated 'look after the stuff' mum. Her family were army barmy, running off into the sea with paddle, surf boards, across the sand with kites. Annemarie was left watching 'the stuff'.

Her mission was to keep up with her family. Her motivation was that she was fed up being the one left out. She was not fit enough. She couldn't join in. She was left out. Annemarie changed all that, you can see her testimonial on my Get Gorgeous website, along with all the other gorgeous girls I have had the divine pleasure of working with.

Perhaps you want that gorgeous pair of jeans that has been sitting in the cupboard for 10 years to fit? Regain your former sexy glory? Maybe it is something a little darker, a lifestyle disease that your parents have succumbed to? "Not like my mum" was Susan's password for her Get Gorgeous website login.

Knowing your why and digging deep helps to make the mindset shift a non-issue. Writing about it, journaling and discussing your thoughts will give you clarity. Spend the time on this part of your journey. The more time and effort you spend on this, the more you will refer back to it, be inspired and re-engage. Register your book, using the code or website reference at the back of this book, I will send you a 'know your why' big picture plan.

Don't change everything at once

Daily habits are added into your day and change your life simply and forever. You are what you do repeatedly. Exercise is not an act but a habit. To paraphrase Aristotle, "We are what we repeatedly do, excellence then is not an act but a habit." My phrase is simplier #justsaying.

Keeping your habits small makes it easier to adopt and keep them. Zorro's circle describes small tasks and working on your small area of competence. Draw a Zorro circle in the sand and concentrate on the small habit that you can achieve. [14]

Task one of the gorgeous principles is stick to water – join the water challenge on my website www.get-gorgeous. com/healthy-tools and feel the benefits of a big personal win. Remember how it made Susan feel: her first win after her hubby died changed her life's direction.

Maintain your happy disposition

Gratitude is the simple solution to maintaining your happy state.

EXERCISE

Three gratitudes every morning and evening.

While your brain is still a little sleepy and you haven't regained full left-brain, analytical consciousness, you are still in the alpha state of daydreaming brainwaves. When you are lulled and working from a different level of awareness, think about and recite three gratitudes each morning and night, different ones each time. Holding your brain in that gratitude awareness will allow your brain to focus on what you want in the future – future thinking.

Don't take yourself too seriously. Rule number 7, which I mentioned in my introduction, came from a book my daughter's music teacher advised me to read. Zander is a music conductor who knows about managing people and getting the best from them, and how to be a good leader. His book, which has a musical, pleasing style, describes how to lead from the back row: each violinist needs to play as if they have the solo spot and as a leader. He also awards an A to all his students, reasoning that it will make them confident and relaxed. They have already achieved what they set out to do. Learning a new piece of music or a new piece of tech in a relaxed fashion is easy, no pressure. You've already got your A. A relaxed learner is a happy learner and will absorb so much more material with a relaxed disposition. [15]

Rule number 7 resonated deeply. Don't take yourself too seriously; enjoy the journey. Be a good learner and watch with interest your hiccups. Another insightful point from the charismatic Zander is to treat each mistake with curiosity. Declare, "That is interesting." It immediately takes the pressure off and allows you to sit back and view how to move forward. I ate that entire bar of Dairy Milk – how curious? Coming from a place of curiosity rather than blame helps to go back and try again. You can commit to a habit when you know you haven't got to start from the beginning each time; setbacks are normal and release the pressure valve.

Habits are created from commitment

Motivation is a very thin and not a very predictable human resource. As discussed previously, it is like a smartphone that needs recharging every night. Every morning you have 100% motivation and you are raring to go. Therefore, exercise in the morning and capitalise on this motivation. Normal everyday choices throughout your day will drain your commitment battery.

It isn't always food choices; it can be something as simple as which shoes to wear. Which direction will be quicker to get to work? Which strategy to follow when implementing Fred's email? You can't fight and push your motivation forward, your inner teenager will rise up and scream, "Ice cream now!"

Successful habits have a strategy

1. Don't overwhelm yourself; adapt and focus on one habit at a time.

2. Be open-minded and remember, "I know, I know," from Robert Cialdini and the mental shortcut that allows us to filter spam from our lives.

3. Relax and be curious about hiccups on your journey.

4. Know your triggers – being bored, lacking time, feeling stressed, feeling scared.

5. Manage your expectations. Success is measured not in a straight diagonal line up, but a very messy, squiggly one.

6. Habits are formed through commitment, not willpower – show up.

7. Use the 90/10 rule: chillax and invoke Rule number 7.

CHAPTER 4

Step into your guiding spirit

Follow your bliss and Ask – Believe – Receive. This chapter covers the cosmic, woo-woo approach to weight loss and ultimate health. Ask, believe and receive is a law of attraction statement and belief structure. What is fascinating is that you can use this approach towards your health.

For example, if you want radiating skin you can receive it. Look up to the warm sun and imagine your skin glowing with health. Wherever you direct your thoughts, your body will follow. Or put simply, imagine that you can relieve headaches by cooling and re-directing the flow of your blood.

When trying to get to sleep, Tracey was always struggling with her brain racing, mind chatter and monkeys and chimps jumping up and down with the thoughts of the day. Visualising her blood being diverted from the area of her headache to elsewhere worked beautifully. She knew it worked and she recovered from 18 months of low-grade migraines her GP had described as menopause-related, which were affecting her sleep. OK, it wasn't Tracey, it is me! Simply focusing my thoughts on the blood flow in my head, channelling away from my frontal lobes which were hot, I could visualise the blood cooling and moving through. It works.

Mind affects body – body affects mind

Your body responds to your thoughts. Natural strong positive emotions rewire your brain. As described earlier, scientists now know that your brain has amazing regenerative capacity, and studies show that you can repair a damaged brain and repair your body – this is called neurogenesis. [1]

Gene mapping has allowed scientists to understand that your environment plays a much more important part in your future and it is possible to turn on and off genes that you once believed your ancestry dictated. Ten years ago, scientists believed that your future was predetermined by your forebears. What a sad, depressing state of affairs, no way out. Your destiny is predetermined. More recently scientists have learned that environment and lifestyle have a huge effect on your ability to switch on and off certain gene predispositions, which is great news for optimists like me. [2]

Thoughts produce chemicals in your brain called neurotransmitters, including serotonin and dopamine, which you may have heard described as the 'happy hormones'. When you think a thought, neurotransmitters are released from one neurone and jump over to another neurone using a bolt of energy or electricity: this is called 'firing'. When you repeat the same thought, you fire off lots of neurones, creating a pattern. Your body then simulates the production of another chemical, which makes its way to the centre of the neurone (the nucleus) and activates several genes of DNA. Therefore, repeated positive thinking creates new connections between neurones, your neural pathway, your mindset and your neurosignature. Boom!

Being positively happy and shining bright will change your gene DNA. Your gene predisposition will be altered. You have a vested interest in seeing the best in life.

What is incredibly exciting is that your change in lifestyle and attitude can effect change in your body and any 'bad' genes that you may have inherited don't have to be activated.

Stem cells are clever little cells than can be created into anything your body desires and think about. Biochemists know that stem cells morph into any type of cells; they have only a stem and thus are able to grow another head, so it could become a bone cell, an immune cell, a skin or heart cell. As genes are activated, the stem cells grow into the cells that they are required to become. Your thoughts can direct your stem cell production. [3]

Claiming your experiences, taking responsibility and owning your day, uplifting your thoughts and becoming positive about your health and feeling powerfully emotional about these events will change your gene profile and create the cells you need to change your health. Big jump? Why not? I am prepared to be very positive and see if it works.

Guided by your higher self

If you and I make the jump that our body will develop and change according to our thoughts, we need to be careful about guiding our thoughts. How do you speak and work with your higher self and your intuition?

By simply listening to the unspoken messages that you feel within your body. Listen to your intuitive self and be guided by your thoughts, intuition and your gut. You will learn more in Chapter 6 that your gut houses two-thirds of your immune system and your hormones are produced there. It is where your true 'gut' instinct originates. In relation to physical exercise, practitioners like Joseph Pilates outline the importance of your powerhouse and the 'core' as the seat of your emotions. This is explored further in Chapter 8.

It is hugely exciting to think that physical exercise, gene knowledge and even nutritional science are all converging and making the same point. Look after your gut, it is the seat of your immunity and your inner thinking. Trust your gut.

Listening to your true nature and speaking your truth impeccably and with integrity means speaking up for yourself and knowing your truth. Speak your instinctive truth in a joyful way and your health will reap the benefits.

At any moment you can ask what would you rather be feeling. Are you trapped in a vicious circle of resentment with a neighbour, friend or partner, perhaps about the cars parked on your street or bins not being cleared up? Or are you looking to find the best in your day, gazing up to the sky to find the blue and taking a few moments to change your DNA? I appreciate that this sounds a little wild and wacky, but the truth is that scientists have no concrete ideas about how our thoughts affect our body, but many are curious, and it is worth exploring.

Your insights and understanding about your body will come from your instincts, so allow them to flow. As a Chinese proverb suggests, write them down: "A thought won't last as long as the faintest of ink." Write down your insights and your thoughts, and hear what you have to say. Your insights are the key to knowing yourself and will allow you to move past your blocks and previous setbacks.

Your body in balance

Your body has the most amazing ability to reset and heal. Your crazy, mad sympathetic nervous system – which is the 'fright, flight or fight' system – is beautifully countered and balanced by the 'rest and digest' parasympathetic nervous system. Your inner teenager runs on your sympathetic nervous system, while your higher self comes from a place where the parasympathetic nervous system resides.

Your sympathetic nervous system – 'fright, flight or fight' – can hijack your emotions. The drama of certain high-energy emotions can overwhelm and take over your thought processes and you become emotionally blinded. Road rage can flare up and you can either fight the car driver, ignore them or ignore your emotions or stay still and stare like a bunny in headlights. These responses are instinctive, primal and part of who you are. You can't avoid your emotions, but you can watch them with interest without reacting.

Your emotions can soar to a high level of intensity, partly because your previous mindset has been triggered. Your emotions are heightened by the thoughts that you put into your processing system, your brain in the past.

When you make yourself aware of your past mindset issues – for instance, you used to believe that all osteopaths were crazy because of something you read in the *Daily Mail* about an osteopathic treatment causing bloodshot eyes – you can register where that belief came from, and then you have the opportunity to view your thoughts and decide how to act.

Some mindsets are easy to spot and change, while others can be more fixed or even permanent. For instance, some of your thoughts come from permanent fixtures based on your value system. Value systems are much harder to identify because they have become part of how you are.

A classic value system could entail something like, "Women work harder than men," or "Honesty and integrity is a value system that is important to me." Others can be based on your religious or spiritual faith.

Other thoughts are more malleable, like software updates, and can be removed and updated. For instance, I thought I needed to do everything in the house, and yet I am not superwoman, I can't do it all. Reframing and updating your brain software is possible. [4]

The purpose of this book is to shift a few of the software updates by calling them out, recognising them as blocks and offering you the opportunity to navigate your way around them. Common health blocks that are in people's software computer programming include:

- I have always been fat.

- *Daily Mail* insights abound: "bloodshot eyes result of osteopath visit." Don't visit an osteopath: they are dangerous.

- My husband won't support me.

- I am a runner; I can't do Pilates that will stretch my muscles and my muscles need to be short to run effectively.

- My genes make me fat.

- I only eat egg whites.

- I can't run.

- Cheese has 8 points and is a matchbox size.

- Exercise in a gym three times a week is enough to keep me healthy.

- The cereals are in the house for my kids.

These thoughts create a drama, a self-fulfilling prophecy. They are keeping you stuck and in paralysis. You are now aware that you can change anything about you, including the limiting statements that you have used to keep you safe. Recognising your limiting statements and linking them will aid your recovery and drive you forward.

Access your inner goddess

In times of stress and indecision, your inner teenager or inner Horace (her borrowed name, so she is easier to identify) will love to take over. When motivation is low, and stress is high, Horace will want to reach for the wine, crisps and cake. It is an instant stress buster, or so it seems.

Looking to the future can be difficult in moments of perceived calamity, but pondering the bigger picture will help divert you from the sugar hangover. Ask your inner goddess for direction.

Asking questions constitutes a simple habit interruption strategy that will give your inner guide a chance to speak up and help you to consider changing your actions.

Questions like:

"What would I rather be experiencing?"

"What action would help me to create my vision?"

If those questions feel too big and maybe too much of a stretch, break them down and look for internal guidance. Linking to your higher self will give you support and guided intuition.

Your neocortex, as previously discussed, is the newest part of your brain and is a slow thinker. She is contemplative, speaks the truth, assesses a situation and offers sound advice. She can be affected by your computer programming, but she also has the innate ability to disentangle the messages, if you give her space. Rest and digest is her best place to be heard. Your inner goddess resides here, she is comfortable sitting back and watching what is going on in your emotions; she is able to guide you if you simply give her space to think. Asking yourself questions prompts her and gives your higher intuition the space to be heard.

What would you rather be feeling?

Centring yourself and coming from a heartfelt place allows you to speak to your higher self. You can be guided and nurtured in your actions by your guiding spirit. Accessing your inner guide with a habit interruption strategy, such as posing a simple question, gives you space to find her.

Access your guide, your inner intuition by using centring tools based on your emotions.

Recognise your guide

You can recognise your guide via your emotional state. For example, when working with clients I find out how they see the world, what type of learners they are. Gorgeous Suzi is a colour expert; she sees colour in her everyday life; her business is based on colour. She is amazing at coordinating her clothing and accessories. Suzi is able to access her guide using colour. When she feels in flow with her creativity and her work, she can feel into a creative emotional state to which she associates a colour. When she sees that colour in her mind's eye, she then knows she is in flow. She is in tune with her inner guidance system. Suzi becomes aware of the presence of her inner guide when that familiar colour comes to her mind.

Another client, Steph, is guided by her physical body. She uses kinesiology to feel a response from her body. Her body gives her access to her inner knowing. For example, she stands tall with great posture and asks herself a question, with her eyes closed, and allows her body to respond.

She sets the intention: 'yes' is forwards and 'no' is backwards. Closing her eyes, she asks a simple question, such as, "Is my name Steph?" Her body responds accordingly, and she knows she is in flow, so she can move on to more difficult questions, such as, "Is it appropriate for me to run today?" or "Should I drink at the party this evening?" Even work questions can be answered in this way, "Should I be working with Joe Wilson with this project?"

Jenny is a fantastic visualiser: she can 'see' her vision. Her inner vision is clear and guides her to the correct course of action. She can see the bigger picture and works towards it; her actions are created because of her goal in life.

Listen to your heart messages

Other insights into your inner guide include experiencing a lightness of body, or a feeling of exhilaration, tears or goose bumps. These will inform you that you are on the right track, that this is the right path for you now.

Centring heart tools are a wonderful way of connecting to your source. Listening to your heart rhythm, watching your heart focus and calm breathing will aid your path to your inner mentor. Our messages so often come from our head, inner teenagers rage when the head responds to an external output. Taking the time to listen to your heart, opening up and noticing how your heart responds is much more intuitive and less destructive.

'Don't knows' are clues

In my coaching practice, I listen to a lot of 'I don't knows'. "How does that make you feel?" "I don't know." "Does that way of behaving upset you?" "I don't know."

Listen for your 'don't knows': they are a clue, an insight into unprocessed emotions. They are a trigger that you can follow up with, if you allow yourself the time to explore. They are a clue that you haven't spent the time noticing your emotions or how you feel about something.

Harness your spiritual to guide your actions.

Once you are in tune with your heart messages, you will quickly recognise what positive or negative experience you are encountering. If something is asked of you and your head says, "I should do that," but your heart is tired and weepy, then you are ignoring your body's emotional state and at some stage you will try and soothe that pain with booze, chocolate, gossip or trashy telly – or even all four at the same time.

Psychologists and human behaviourists talk about motivating your elephant, meaning your emotions, and directing your rider, which refers to your brain. Another way of looking at your inner world is in terms of your rational thinking rider and your emotional elephant. [5]

Your rider may have a good idea for your future; she might be jumping up and down in excitement about reaching a size 8 in the six-week 'eat nothing' bikini diet. Your rational rider knows that may not be possible, but if you get up at 6am, run every day, drop *all* carbs, snack on 1g of lettuce, fast every other day *then maybe* you will reach your goal. The rider uses bright spots analogy and has noticed what has worked for others.

Your elephant, however, may have other goals that don't include lettuce. Your elephant is 6t worth of grey matter and isn't so easily moved by the rider, who is a little overenthusiastic and slightly barmy. Your rider offers the direction you want and if she is clever enough, she can outsmart your emotions, but your elephant is slower and needs more time. She also needs a strong emotional draw. She needs to feel motivated and on board. Your emotional elephant needs to feel self-confident about the goal. "Is this goal realistic? Am I going to fail again?" If your emotional elephant isn't feeling confident, then she won't have the motivation to even get started, let along chomp on lettuce every day.

Riders follow a logical part of your brain and use your backlog of computer evidence to figure out what has worked for you in the past, or others that have a successful approach. It is why Instagram does well with before-and-after stories. Our riders climb on board, yeah! I can do that. The rider can see the vision and believes it can work for them.

Elephants need a lot of emotional convincing. I think the elephant analogy is good – she is weighty and substantial, and she needs a lot to move and motivate her, but she is also the successful, deep thinker. However, I feel a tad uncomfortable thinking about weight loss and elephants in the same sentence, not good for morale. How about the emotional elephant being like a graceful hot air balloon? Once she is filled up with motivation, she will easily fly above the daily drudge. Emotional elephants are your higher self, or in terms of neuroscience the neocortex part of the brain. The slow thinker, but once motivated will fly. Visualise elephants in a hot air balloon of 'confidence'.

Pathway to success

Getting involved emotionally in your outcome will shape your path to success. Action triggers can get things moving, as discussed earlier, like exercising early in the morning before your brain has woken up and before your motivation cup has been drained by your decision-making day. Preplanning your week, food planning as Joe Wicks calls it, "prepping like a boss" and diarising your exercise. I do mean putting your exercise in your diary. I spend time with some clients and work out when they can get out in the fresh air and walk, or the best time of day to work out with my Gorgeous Pilates or aerobics membership site videos.

Once you have your emotions on board, navigate your own path and lay out your plan, which is a requisite: life is too busy not to have a plan. A plan will help the obliger tendencies in you. I have a plan, which has to be followed; the more you follow the plan the harder it is to leave the plan. Another word for plan is habit. Your plan will quickly become a habit and habits are very hard to break.

Get your friends on board

We've talked about having like-minded friends: being with harmonious, enthusiastic, healthy eating, and focused individuals will have an effect on you. Getting your friends on board with your lifestyle will help you. Simply put, rally your girlfriend herd.

Chris, a physiotherapist who attends my Pilates classes (and features on my YouTube channel), explained an example of 'rallying the herd', which I adored. Chris and her friends meet three times a year. They all come from different parts of the country and it is often difficult to organise diary dates, but they persevere and set aside a weekend together. Not as you might imagine to drink and sit by open fires and catch up. They met as walking friends, so now they meet for walking weekends, covering up to 35 miles over a weekend. They enjoy the countryside in various counties around the country and stay fit. That is my kind of friendship. Behaviour is contagious, and Chris's friends are all motivated by each other.

Like-minded people. Following a crowd and moving towards where you want to go is easier when you move towards the group of people who are already portraying the attributes that you want. This is a common business practice – you don't want to be the brightest person in the room, you want to be the least experienced, with the most to learn, then you can absorb from the other shining stars.

Your social grouping can be categorised into two different personality types: radiators and drainers. Those in life that offer you warmth and empathy and the drainers that suck the life out of you – I like the 'dementor' imagery. It is graphic.

What about those friends that you need a social connection with, but not a big emotional investment – those five-minute dog-walking friendships or the local shopkeeper, who you want to acknowledge, say hi but don't have much in common with, or the next door neighbour who is a half-an-hour friend? Those friends who you want to cultivate and enjoy are two-day friendships or longer. Noticing where you spend your energy and on whom is an important part of your health. Bear in mind that whether everyone cares for your way of life or your views is not your concern. What others think of you is none of your business. That is easier said than done, but when you are clear-headed it becomes easier; ignore life's 'trolls' and focus on your goals. [6]

"Ignore life's trolls and focus on your goals." @adelestickland – you can TWEET that one ;-)

EXERCISE

List five 'dementors' in your life, those individuals who drain you.

List five radiators in your life, those friends and family members who lift you.

Believe in yourself: you are amazingly gorgeous

Life experiences and people create an emotional static that can weigh you down and put you off your game. Future thinking and feeling into your vision will pave your way to your successful healthy vision of your future. Practising feeling your emotion and putting a vision in place will allow your neurones to fire up and pull you towards your goal. You will 'see' opportunities that will bring you closer to your goal.

CHAPTER 5

Caring for yourself is your duty

Developing a sense of self and who you really are can be surprisingly difficult, especially for women. You are probably unaware that you haven't got a strong sense of identity. Realistically, what we do is tied up with other people's needs and wants – including paying a mortgage and listening to your boss, your customers, the people and animals in your life you care for. Who are you among all those roles?

Neurolinguistic programming (NLP) describes your personality as a way of surviving childhood. Your personality develops according to who you need to be to best fit into your family dynamic. Ask my sister about middle child syndrome: she will give you a detailed account. Growing up as the oldest sister, I created a responsible (some would say bossy) manner, which seems to serve me well as a Pilates instructor and health coach.

The real you is hidden under layers of social and family conditioning. Authors outline this in a cyclical manner that can evolve in seven-year cycles. [1]

Your emotional hardwiring, your computer, has imprints even before you're born. *In utero*, you experience your mother's feelings and emotions as she does. You are aware of her vibrations and her happiness and sorrow through her hormones, which flow into your bloodstream. Your mother's feelings of security and happiness are recorded by you emotionally even before your birth. If she happens to have had a difficult pregnancy, with work stresses, money issues or a relationship break-up, this is emotionally reflected in your life. You may have a feeling of abandonment or money scarcity issues that can reflect throughout your life. You are not conscious of these events or their recurring theme. You didn't even know they were there, because they are based on something that isn't in your conscious thought. They are an emotional hangover from your ancestral line, societal thinking, such as a Protestant work ethic, or an emotion that occurred when you were too young to remember.

Why does this keep happening to me?

From the ages birth to seven, you are an emotional child. You understand the world through your emotions; everything is either hugely exciting or massively disappointing. If at this tender age your dad loses his job, or your parents get divorced, you have an imprinted feeling of this event. You may feel needy and abandoned or feel money scarcity in stages throughout your life.

Later on, between the ages of seven and 14, your influences at school are varied. Your emotions are heightened in your teenage years, and there is an imperative to be accepted by the herd. At school, your brain is taking on a lot about 'how to behave' in society, and a lot of activity is mental and cerebral, with the processing of new information. If, at this time, your best friend moves away from school, which for some would not be an issue, but is for you due to your earlier experiences, it has more significance.

The adult world feels physical. You are aware of the world and what is going on around you, how to get on in your career, what your car or holidays look like. Your internal world is less important and paying attention to your feelings becomes subordinate. If at the age of 20 a relationship breaks off, this can simply fuel your abandonment story. Or if your pension loses value, it adds to your 'money scarcity' belief.

These incidents may have occurred to other people in a similar way, but their effect on their self-confidence is not the same.

We all have untold, unnoticed stories that don't need to be uncovered and systematically reviewed. Simply be aware of how you react to your triggers, people or situations. Look at your emotional reactions to a situation. The feeling of being bullied is an emotional trigger for me. If I feel that someone is pushing me or overriding me, the 'small person trigger' in me pops up. I think I am aware of it and I look after myself and review the situation asap to ensure that 'small person trigger' mode doesn't go awry.

If you are unaware of these triggers, or miss the cycle, you can become emotionally blind to situations and the "Why does this keep happening to me?" feeling resurfaces. Until you, gorgeous girl, take responsibility.

Being 'emotionally blind' to your needs means that you may use drama to get attention from others, because you may not be emotionally aware enough to know how to give yourself love and compassion. This drama can manifest in overreacting, eating too much, working too hard or even over-exercising. [2]

Hang ups stem from unprocessed feelings

Instead of noticing or expressing feelings, we can use a number of destructive patterns, like eating over our feelings, drinking over them, working over them, using drugs, gossiping or simply complaining over them.

EXERCISE [3]

Practise describing a feeling.

Feel it for 90 seconds and feel it change naturally.

Allow it to pass through you naturally.

Past feelings are safe to experience.

Honour them and release them.

As a child, you are full of enthusiasm about life. If we no longer express our feelings, it can repress our frustrations, even our enthusiasm for life, which will have a long-term effect on our lives. Finding peace with yourself and your self is guided by your heart. Your heart provides a clue to your emotions; your mental activity forms your thoughts and this is reflected back to your physical being.

Which brings me on to the subject once again of the law of attraction and quantum physics. Newtonian laws of physics held that matter and cells were stationary, that you could look into a cell and the nucleus would be in the centre and electrons flying around. It is what kids are still taught in school. We now know that, however, as 'observer bias'. Simply put, when a scientist looked inside a cell using a microscope it affected the activity within that cell.

With technology, scientists can now appreciate that inside every cell is simply matter – empty space. Within every cell of your body there is no solid or anything static; it is simply energy. Everything that is alive, no matter how solid it appears to us, is alive and in constant movement. Newborn babies are aware and conscious of the energy that surrounds them, and they have to struggle focusing on the physical world because energies are moving in front of them.

As we grow, we lose the ability to see energy because we have become used to the physical world and what we can see. If this is too big a 'woo-woo' step, just know that science and psychotherapy are beginning to overlap. If energy in the world of science is simply matter that can be transferred through emotions, you can pick up on other people's emotions, and once you have awareness of your emotions, you can create a very different future for yourself.

Put yourself at the centre of your life

Thinking of yourself can feel selfish and strange. However, by not listening to your emotions and being aware of your 'state' of feelings then you are not able to serve those that you adore and want to help. It is a fundamental shift in the way you relate to who you are and what you do in life.

Circumstances don't dictate your success

Previously we have discussed 'blocks' or old stories that you have told yourself about why you can't lose weight or why you are unhealthy. We have talked through how this keeps your mindset fixed and how this creates a neurosignature. Unblocking comes from changing your outlook on life and science backs up the law of attraction and the quantum physical belief that everything is energy. You can therefore attract energy into your life, but which type, positive or negative, is down to you. Therefore, focusing on yourself and the way you speak to yourself is the start of this process. Hence the chapter heading – caring for yourself is your duty. You are creating the world that you know.

Limiting beliefs about yourself will perpetuate the life that exists for you currently. Limiting yourself comes from believing what others say about or to you. When you are unable or unwilling to stand up for yourself and when you don't follow through with your convictions, a little bit of you is lost. If you carry the persecution complex that everybody is looking down on you, then you will seek the opportunities for people to look down on you.

If you look for the positive in people, the pieces of gold that everyone you meet has to offer, then you will indeed find gold in every situation and everyone.

On the other hand, if you feel inferior or unworthy, a hidden, limiting belief or 'imposter syndrome' can become a low-level energy drain. It is a background noise, or a computer software system, whirring in the background, draining your resources. Limiting statements or beliefs such as, "I could never to do that," is an example of this limiting belief, as is, "Thank goodness you don't know the real me."

Developing your sense of self

The relationship you cultivate with yourself is the most important relationship in your life. The relationship with yourself will reflect and bounce back in the relationship you have with your loved ones.

For example, Lorraine had a successful career as a Hong Kong stock market trader. She earned a lot of money and was brilliant at her job. It was a high-stress, high-earning and high-burn-out role. What a blast. When her older sister became ill, went through a painful divorce and found her life too difficult to manage, she and her three daughters and two dogs all moved in with Lorraine. Lorraine went to work in a high-flying, cortisol-revved environment and came home to more drama and upset. Over some years when life changed, Lorraine moved to a different country, and life settled down. Her sister remarried and moved away. Life was good.

Lorraine life's changed beyond recognition. She had a new job, with regular hours and fewer obligations, but she kept her stress. Stress was still in everything she did. Getting dressed in the morning and going to work was a daily drama, fraught with anxiety. Lorraine's relationships with her own daughters, dog and husband were fraught. Control was the main driver, doing everything for her girls including brushing their hair, tying up their shoelaces, making dinners, beds and lunches, as well as working full time. She was still very busy and exasperated. "I never thought being a mum would be like this," she said. Lorraine is the most caring, kind-natured, beautiful woman and yet even the smallest of tasks creates the biggest of issues. Lorraine has ignored herself and focused on others, with a huge heart, but to the great detriment of herself and her new family.

Working with Lorraine to see the stress pattern that she had created enabled her to work towards a calmer future. Her insights have changed her stress levels, she attends a yoga class and practises meditation using a phone app, to and from work. As we worked together, she made small changes that have helped enormously with her sense of wellbeing, she has lost a huge amount of weight, but more importantly she has regained her sense of calm and peace.

Loving yourself must be a daily practice

Cultivating your sense of self includes cultivating self-esteem, self-confidence and your self-belief. These are the cornerstones to loving yourself; putting yourself first each day will reflect back on everyone in your life and everything you do.

Self-esteem is the value you put on yourself. How do you take compliments? Do you deflect or honour them and say thank you?

Self-confidence comes from trusting yourself, being true to your word, keeping your promises to yourself. If you decide that you are going to eat well, then work out your goals and stick to your promises to yourself. Each time you break a promise to yourself, you erode your own self-confidence. You won't feel you can rely on yourself and it will affect your self-esteem. Boosting other people's confidence is the quickest way to improve your own. Complimenting others, seeing the gold in every relationship, will enhance your own self-confidence.

Self-belief is the faith that you have in your abilities. If you were congratulated for your hard work as a child, rather than your attainment, you will have a belief system that you are capable and have the ability to get the job done. John McEnroe is a famous example of somebody with low self-esteem. In his biography, he explains his tennis outbursts. He was always the best. At tennis school he was the best; he rocked. He could do no wrong. He was always acknowledged as the one having reached the highest standard. When you are told you are the best throughout your early years, you believe it. When you are praised for attainment rather than practice, it is a very long fall to the floor.

Kids in school are praised for their effort. Effort and practice reaches goals. Basketball star Michael Jordan practises constantly to maintain his prestigious career. Golfing pro Tiger Woods has the same mental strength, practising and creating the successful edge through hard work, not relying on ability. Success comes from 10% skill and 90% effort and the self-belief that you have the strength of character to last.

EXERCISE

Five things you like about yourself.

When I introduce this exercise in workshops,
it is the hardest for the participants to do. Working
out who their five radiators and dementors are —
is easy. Looking inward and finding your own
gold takes practice.

Do you suffer from 'empty cup' syndrome?

Being busy is a badge of honour women wear with pride. The headspace mind chatter runs around a bit like this: "I am running around after everybody else. I am very busy, busy, very busy. Therefore I am loved because people need me."

And yet, you can't pour from an empty cup, which has become my mantra when working with clients. What does looking after everyone else give you? Psychologists know you can't change behaviour if the situation currently serves you in some way. If the situation supports a feeling that you are needed and loved by being busy and looking after others, then you will never turn your attention to yourself. Loving yourself is much harder than loving other people. We can forgive other people's mistakes, but our transgressions are a little harder to let go of. Reference table dancing in pubs!

If you feel that being needed by someone is more important than your own health, you will never focus on yourself. You are trapped in your own lack of self-esteem bubble. Guilt is huge in our society. Whether that is work guilt, or parent guilt, it is prevalent.

Victorian kids used to be ignored in the corner and even up to the last two generations a well-spoken, well-behaved child was applauded. We know now that children's needs and experiences need to be understood and discussed openly. However, the pendulum has swung the other way. Children are now the centre of most people's universe; they have the control. They can dictate what they eat, when and what they perceive their needs to be, without the experience of maturity. Kids are materially given as much as every parent can afford, but children lack the skills to manage their own lives and emotions.

Mothers' guilt has exploded within our work culture. The last century of motherhood has shaped our version of motherhood today, and yet we have no chance of matching it. I can't bake a cake and run two businesses. If I am really honest, I don't want to bake cakes, yet my daughter would love me to. I have given her the books, YouTube and Mary Berry, who is everyone's grandmother. Modern communication means that celebrities can fill the gaps. Phew! Google was created for a reason.

As a classic latchkey kid from the 1980s, I lived in a broken home where cooking was not a prerequisite skill. My mum was a computer system analyst at a time when the world of tech was run by young men. She couldn't tell anyone she had kids at home; it would have affected her career chances. Whether that was perception or reality is an interesting question.

Parents from the previous generation were generally stay-at-home mums, with little or no office or paid work. If they did work, they were persecuted or demonised for it. Mums today have the pleasure of demonising themselves. You know that you don't need to have it all, but we still try and look like we can.

Emancipated kids and 'pink gene' husbands

Give your family, your nearest and dearest the opportunity to step in and step up. Prepare your kids for the big life beyond the family by encouraging them to make their own eggs in the morning. This means freeing you up, plus it gives them the freedom they crave and need to fulfil their own sense of self. A prerequisite added to my wedding vows included, "You will cook a better roast dinner than me."

Keep your power

Habit interruption strategies are an excellent way of talking to and attracting the attention of your inner goddess. Wait before you say yes to the next request of your time. Count to five and breathe then answer. Or perhaps ask yourself the question, "Do I want to do this?" and wait for your heart to answer. Or simply repeating the question back to the petitioner is an incredibly powerful tool, "You would like me to write that report by 5pm this evening?"

Be more like curious George, be interested in your response to a request of your time. What is your immediate reaction and what is your secondary reaction? Notice the speed of your delivery. When something goes wrong and you end up accepting an impossibly quick deadline, instead stop, breathe and be more like Mr Zander the orchestra conductor, "That is interesting. Why did I behave like that?" Avoid the blame frame. If you say yes, it is not the recipient's fault. Take responsibility and step into your own growth.

Identify your health blind spots

Are you always in a rush, too busy to think and unable to ask for help? Find some free, healthy rituals – #selfcaresunday, baths, walking. Create a habit that is free. For instance, replace pizza Friday with #facemaskFriday; replace wine Friday with #nowineFriday and #exerciseSaturday. Experiment with what works for you and your family.

Record how you feel about self-care Sunday – all emotions are interesting and offer a clue to your ancestral, work ethic parental cueing. Revisit your plans and enjoy new experiences.

Slow down and you will be more creative

Recent research at Cambridge University assessed the validity of being bored and how it is of benefit to you. MRI [magnetic resonance imaging] scanning of the brain has shown that while being bored your brain is actually piecing your day together. The research suggests that downing a gear is essential for your health.

Cambridge University's speculative conclusion was that being bored leads to the stimulation of creativity, productivity and fulfilment in your life. Using MRI brain scans, researchers monitored participants while they were learning a new game of cards. There was a substantial amount of brain activity. The activity in these particular areas of the brain diminished when the game became easier. [4]

However, when the game became easier and the participants became bored – which was described as periods of inactivity – the brain scans lit up in different areas, not in the areas where new experiences were stimulated. The researchers found that the brain was still highly active while in a non-learning state. Boredom seemed to take as much effort as actively doing something. The brain is highly active in the background, even when it is not carrying out any specific tasks.

They concluded that valuable behaviours such as creativity increase when your brain is idle. While unproductive the brain may be processing and filing life's daily experience, allowing your brain space to catalogue new information.

Relaxation is countercultural

Be a rebel and be bored. Socrates the Greek advised that a life of contemplation was the life of richness and creativity. The Romans debated whether life should be 'active' or 'contemplative'.

In the last 500 years, we have been driven by a Protestant work ethic, no room for debate. Debate over. Being idle is regarded as a sin. And yet boredom increases productivity. Research from refugee camps where enforced boredom was rife showed that once the opportunity presented itself to be busy, entrepreneurial activity accelerated. Being bored makes you more productive. Give yourself some space to think and find creative solutions to mindset blocks. Socrates was right on the money, religion not so much. [5]

The life of activity is the current societal norm. The 'Protestant work ethic' has led to our modern 'always working' culture in which idleness is scorned. Protestant thinking is that contemplation is sinful. Resting and digesting is currently deemed countercultural.

Technology is making us more impatient

While new technology that saves us time is constantly being introduced, the time saved is spent doing more and more things, so our lives are faster paced and more hectic than ever. Apparently most of us are checking our smartphones nine times or more a day. Those little spaces of 'no work', such as walking through a park, are disappearing. You can even work while walking to work!

And with that pendulum swing of history, once we go too far, the pendulum swings back. There is an increasing appreciation of various modes of doing less. You can see this with the increase on alternative therapies, an explosion of coffee shops and the expansion of the leisure industry, as people realise that you have to make the effort to do nothing.

'Downtime' is an essential part of brain activity that helps us to reason with ourselves, and is needed to process life emotions and experiences, and to aid creativity and better thinking.

When you fall asleep at night, your filing system takes over. The day is processed and catalogued. If you meditate or take time during your day to rest and digest, your brain can carry out this processing then, rather than when you want to go to sleep. If you have had a busy day, then there are more things to file, store and categorise. It is natural and, as explained previously, you can't stop these thoughts – you can only watch with interest. Investing in downtime is a habit that needs to be managed and cultivated.

Spending time unwinding will enable you to be more creative, thinking around problems rather than staying stuck within them. Breaking free from the habitual mind loops will allow you freedom to come up with more creative solutions to life dilemmas and daily traumas.

Asking yourself questions is an easy way to break a mind cycle of rinse and repeat. Asking questions of yourself will allow you the opportunity to listen to your inner guidance system, giving yourself that moment to stop and reflect and be open-hearted with yourself and others, rather than feeding the inner teenager the rage she actually wants to let go of.

CHAPTER 6

Your perfect weight

"Weak science, strong personalities, vested interests and political expediency have initiated this series of experiments."

British Medical Journal

We currently have a whirlwind of 'sensational' nutritional thinking. The average person is bombarded with varying facts and distorted research every day.

This section will outline current thinking, in simple terms. It will discuss how scientists and doctors formed their views over the last 50 years, and the research used to create the 'healthy heart diet', which is increasingly being questioned. This section will give you the information you need to make your own informed conclusions.

There is no hype, just plain speaking, and I would like to suggest that if you are prepared to leave your preconceptions behind, follow your instinct and be guided by your inner truth, weight loss is in fact incredibly easy. You can feel and look fantastic every day.

The carb 'hungry cycle'

Let's begin with a simple explanation of the macronutrients: carbohydrates, proteins and fats. Micronutrients are the vitamins and minerals you receive from your food. Calorie counting isn't necessary if you are eating fats and proteins. Carbohydrates, as I will explain later, are the lowest in the calorie spectrum, but they also make you the hungriest and put you in a hungry cycle. If you are eating protein and fats you won't get hungry. It is as simple as that. You can hear the diet world and a few fellow nutritionists screaming at me.

Losing weight and diseases like diabetes, arthritis and even dementia are not multifactorial. There is an interesting similarity between these diseases that is quite straightforward. Occam's razor is the philosophical belief that the simplest answer is generally the right one. The assumption with the least speculation is usually better. The first half of the book was about trusting your inner guidance system for a reason. This chapter explains why.

Understand your macronutrients

Proteins are broken down in your body to form amino acids. There are nine essential amino acids. These amino acids need to be consumed every day, hence the name 'essential'. Protein foods include meat, seafood, eggs, chia seeds, fish and hempseed.

Organic meat contains all nine essential amino acids in one mouthful, as do eggs. Vegetarians and vegans need to select foods that combine to create a complete protein in a slightly different way. I have written a blog and produced a video outlining how to create this . Vegans and vegetarians need to combine protein and carbs to make up the essential amino acids. The easy-to-remember combo is 'grain and pulse' to form a complete vegetarian protein. [1]

Carbs are broken down by your body into glucose, and insulin is instantly released by your body whenever glucose is in circulation. Insulin and glucose are a team and work together. Insulin mops up glucose and feeds it to muscle or liver cells, or panics and puts it into storage – fat storage (also known as love handles).

Carbs are ranked with a score out of 100 on the glycaemic index, a figure representing their relative ability to increase the level of glucose in your blood – the higher the number the quicker your 'carb' hit.

White or beige carbs are bread, oats, fruit, potatoes and green carbs include fruit and vegetables.

Dietary fats are broken down by the body into fatty acids. Fats are also broken down into elements. Foods with *monounsaturated fats* include macadamias, olives and oil, avocado, pecans, almonds, cashews and peanut butter, lard, chicken and duck fat.

Polyunsaturated fats are found in fish (salmon, mackerel), fish oil, Brazil nuts, walnuts, plus seeds like pumpkin, hemp, sunflower, sesame, chia and flaxseeds. Polyunsaturated fats are further broken down into omega-3 and omega-6 fatty acids. These two fatty acids are finely tuned and, like your parasympathetic and sympathetic nervous system, they help to balance your gorgeous body in perfect homeostasis – balance. The balance of omega 3:6 ratio should ideally be 1:1.

Omega-3 is the anti-inflammatory fat and is found in fish, chia seeds and flaxseeds. Walnuts contain a little omega-3 but more omega-6. Omega-6 is the inflammatory fat and is found in vegetable oils: corn, cottonseed, soybean, sunflower, peanut, canola oil and soybean and peanuts. Your body needs both fatty acids to work with each other to create balance.

Unfortunately the typical modern diet has changed beyond recognition in the last 50 years: the amount of omega-6 in our food chain has increased via animal feed, vegetable oils in cooking and processed food so that its ratio to omega-3 is now 6:1, not at a balanced 1:1.

Reduce your risk of dementia

Research published in the *Neurology* journal in 2007 looked at 8,000 participants with normal brain function and four years later found that those individuals who never ate fish had increased their risk of dementia and Alzheimer's by 37%. Those participants who consumed fish every day reduced their risk by 44%. Those participants who ate omega-3 in olive, flaxseed and walnut oil were 60% less likely to develop dementia. Those who consumed high levels of omega-6 in vegetable oils were 50% more likely to develop dementia. Regular users of butter had no significant change in their risk of dementia. [2]

Butter does not increase your dementia (or cardiovascular) risk, but if you do *not* eat fish or other foods containing omega-3 then you have an increased likelihood of dementia. Eating fats from vegetable oils like sunflower oil *increases* your risk of dementia.

TOP TIP

Eating a handful of nuts with avocado is a perfect snack because it combines monounsaturated and polyunsaturated fats.

Saturated fats are found in coconut oil, animal fats and dairy (cheese, milk and cream), eggs, palm oil, soya milk and tofu. Saturated fats have been demonised over the last 50 years, for reasons that are misleading and factually unsound. I will explain this in detail.

TOP TIP

Free 'fat chart' summary when you register your book.

Trans-fatty acids are modern, man-made and deadly. They didn't exist until 50 years ago. They are created through chemical processing, corrupted fats that have been modified and when cooked are lethal. Trans-fatty acids are molecules that have been deformed during a process called hydrogenation.

TOP TIP

Avoid foods with 'hydrogenated vegetable oils'
on their labels.

Most fast-food restaurants cook with trans-fats. It is not their fault, as they were advised by the health bodies to use vegetable oils, the frying of which is causing unmeasured health risks.

Trans-fats are found in shop-bought, manufactured cakes, biscuits, crisps, pies, muffins, pizzas, breads, microwave popcorn, sweets, margarines and cake mix. Trans-fats are also found in manufactured low-fat products. Low-fat foods are low in saturated fat, but high in sugar (although this is being addressed) and in hydrogenated oils, to increase their shelf life.

TOP TIP

Avoid food that doesn't go mouldy in a week.

TOP TIP

Most food cooked in restaurants, especially fast-food restaurants, is cooked in trans-fats to make it tastier. AVOID.

Myth-busting summary

According to research, omega-6 vegetable fats are linked to the risk of dementia. [3] Trans-fats are found in hydrogenated vegetable oils, which are commonly used in fast-food outlets and in processed foods. Trans-fats are used to extend the shelf life of products, and you should avoid food that doesn't go mouldy. To confirm and reconfirm, butter does not increase your risk of dementia or heart disease.

You need to combine your food macronutrients

Current NHS and American heart guidelines advise eating a 'healthy heart' diet based on fruits, vegetables and whole grains with modest portions of lean meat and low-fat dairy produce. Red meat is not represented, nor are full-fat milk, cream cheese and butter. Eggs do not feature prominently either.

Recommendations in the form of the Eat well Plate in the UK and My Plate in USA suggest 60% carbs, 20% fat (type not specified) and 20% protein, whereas your ancestors' diet typically contained 75% fat, 20% protein and 5% carbs. Native Americans who lived a traditional way of life, eating a diet of predominantly meat, mainly from buffalo, and were observed between 1898 and 1905, were apparently "spectacularly healthy and lived to a ripe old age". [4] Vilhjalmur Stefansson, an anthropologist who lived and studied a group of Inuit, observed in 1946 that they consumed between 70% and 80% of their daily energy intake from fat.

Current health statistics in the UK and USA are worrying. Diagnoses of diabetes have tripled in the last 40 years. In the US, cases of diabetes jumped by 50% in 42 states between 1995 and 2010 and there was a 100% increase in 18 states. In 2014, 62% of adults in England were classified as overweight (having a body mass index of 25 or above) or obese. More than two-thirds of men and almost six in 10 women are overweight or obese. [5]

What is even more alarming is that the number of people with Alzheimer's disease is likely to outstrip the number who are obese by 2050, affecting an estimated 100 million people.[6] Alzheimer's disease has been called type 3 diabetes, as the factors associated with cognitive decline and with diabetes appear to be similar.

Fats do not make you fat

The predominance of carbohydrates in the western diet has coincided with an explosion in ill health, of the type that leads to a slow and painful death. "Almost nothing that we commonly believe today about fats generally and saturated fat in particular appears upon close examination to be accurate," wrote Nina Teicholz in *The Big Fat Surprise.*

Nina spent 10 years investigating and systematically reviewing every piece of research, and I consider her to be meticulous and pragmatic. *The Big Fat Surprise* was book of the year in 2014 for the *Times*, *Wall Street Journal* and the *BBC Food Programme*. It was described in the *British Medical Journal* as "a remarkable job in analysing how weak science, strong personalities, vested interests and political expediency have initiated this series of experiments." [7]

How the fat myth began

I appreciate that this is hard to understand for most left-brain thinkers (including me) but the proof really is in the pudding. The fat myth and the healthy heart diet and eating in 'moderation' has been our mantra since birth. I am asking you to try out some new ideas and be flexible in your thinking.

When I first heard from my dear paediatrician friend, back in the early 1990s, that fruit juices were making kids obese, I was extremely upset. I had been serving healthy apple juice to my only son, thinking I was being a great mum. As with any dramatic life event, I can even remember exactly where I was when I was told that: doing a 24-hour charity walk. I was so shocked, confused and angry.

When I started to understand the fat myth or the 'lipid myth', I also remember exactly where I was – reading masses of books and research. The place was different, but the feelings were the same.

During the second world war, Americans and Britons were the healthiest they have ever been, statistically, and this was the case for Americans too during the Great Depression. [8] Some scientists have argued that it was because there was little red meat, while others have attributed it to general scarcity of food. Others have begun to argue that it was because there was a shortage of bread and wheat.

Scientists in Holland noted that schizophrenia and death from coeliac disease dropped significantly during the shortages of the war years. Through systematic analysis and research over a number of years, it eventually led them to believe that modern-day wheat causes huge inflammation in the brain. [9]

The brain has no pain receptors, so you can't tell that you have brain inflammation until you are diagnosed with Alzheimer's disease or another form of dementia. We shall explore this more later.

"No organ is more susceptible to detritus effect of inflammation than the brain."[10] The big question we will cover later is what causes inflammation? The point is neuroscientists, nutritionists and biochemists all noticed that the west was very different before the war years.

Fat myth began ...

After the war, President Eisenhower suffered three heart attacks (while in office). He smoked three packs of cigarettes a day, but at the time doctors were endorsing cigarette smoking, so that was overlooked. [11]

The race was on to find out the culprit for the President's heart attacks. A prominent, very good-looking and charismatic (a lot of assumptions there on my part) Dr Ancel Keys from the University of Minnesota carried out his famous *Seven Countries* study. [12] He looked at the statistical relationship between Japan and USA, because there were proportionately fewer incidents of heart attacks in the Japanese population. The statistics were based on Japanese people consuming 10% of their calories from fat and having a low incidence of coronary artery disease (CAD), while people in the US consumed 40% of their calories from fat and there were high levels of CAD in the population. Interestingly, Japan had a significant increase in the number of strokes suffered during this period, but that was not included in the findings. Dr Keys concluded that animal fats formed a large part of the US diet, but not the Japanese, and that therefore cholesterol gives you a heart attack – he used the word 'lipids' and it all sounded very impressive.

Ancel Keys' *Seven Countries* study ignored France and Germany, whose populations eat a lot of fat – stuffed ducks, pâté, sausage and so forth. These countries were ignored: they didn't fit the results.

A lone UK-based scientist, John Yudkin, a lecturer at University College London (mild-mannered and wore a tweed jacket – again, huge assumptions on my part, just building the picture) explained that it was sugar, not dietary fat, that increased the risk of heart attacks. Yudkin was laughed out of nutritional conferences and ridiculed. His work was disparaged, and in his lifetime he was ignored. (13)

Michael Mosley, a television journalist, producer, presenter and author who is credited with popularising the 5:2 diet, is among the protagonists of Yudkin's work. He recalls from his own experience that his father had a high risk of stroke and heart attack and was placed on the 'heart-healthy' diet. This diet includes 'healthy grains'. Grains (think carbs) when broken down make glucose. Processed

GORGEOUS

grain (carbs) make a lot of glucose. Don't fret: insulin – the
heroine of the hour – mops up the glucose and you return
to normal again. The problems occur, as you know, when
your body is under constant assault from a high-carb diet.
A high-carb diet looks like this:

- cereal or toast for breakfast with fruit juice

- sandwich for lunch

- dinner with rice or potatoes

- snacking on fruit, bread and cereal bars

Unhealthy chocolate bars are deemed to be the culprit for
obesity, when in reality it is the high-carb meals that are
the biggest culprits, and the snacks are overload.

As an astonished GP, Michael watched his father become
fatter on the heart-healthy diet he had been prescribed. [14]
He made the link with sugar, hence his interest in the 5:2
diet and his amazing work advocating the reduction of
sugar and intermittent fasting.

The lipid debate that raged in the 1960s and 70s
continues to feature, despite the fact there has never been
a comprehensive study to prove this link. [15]

Back in the 1950s, the 'prudent' diet was introduced in the
US and the western world replaced butter, lard, eggs and
beef with margarine, corn oil, chicken and cereal. The
'lipid myth' perpetuated throughout the 1970s and billions
of dollars were spent on cholesterol-lowering drugs.

My mum slapped the healthiest thing 'since sliced bread'
on the table in the form of trans-fat margarine: Flora on
our brown bread after we had munched through Weetabix

to which we had added healthy 'brown' sugar because it needed sweetening.

We were ahead of the game in our village, but little did we realise that by following so-called healthy heart guidelines we were right on the button for diabetes, heart attack and dementia.

In the 1980s, fast-food restaurants removed beef tallow from their chips and on the advice of healthy heart specialists. Fast-food restaurants now cook with man-made, synthetically produced trans-fats.

The message still is that fats are bad, carbs are good. "Doctors endorsed smoking with the same kind of ignorance." [16]

In 1994, the American Diabetes Association recommended the current guidelines quoted at the beginning of this chapter: 60-70% calories from carbs. Between 1997 and 2007, the number of diagnoses of diabetes exploded, tripling from 1980 to 2011. [17]

In 1988, the Surgeon General's office decided to gather all the evidence linking saturated fat to heart disease and thus silence the naysayers. In 1999, 11 years later, the office decided that without additional expertise and staff resources they couldn't continue with the study. The study ended because they didn't have the staff to continue it! Or, more honestly, the evidence. They found no evidence to support the 'lipid myth' diet-heart hypothesis. [18]

As things currently stand, nutritional thinking in the medical fraternity does not support the concept of holistic health. This is why you keep getting confusing messages and sensational headlines, such as 'coconut oil is pure poison'. [19]

The false belief that fats make you fat and that cholesterol causes heart attacks, which we have been living with for the last five decades, has become entrenched. For whatever reason, whether that is vested interest or ego or the inability to look at the bigger picture, dissident frustrated voices are being heard in both the US and UK. What began with science researchers and medical journalists has trickled into the arena of fitness and the 'subversive' world of alternative medicine, but hasn't yet hit the mainstream.

On breakfast TV a few months ago, I was horrified to see Trudi Deacon (a respected nutritionist) being treated in condescending manner by a NHS dietician. In a deeply insulting conversation, Trudi's thinking was called 'dangerous' and she was accused of creating panic for the nation because she believes that fats are healthy and eats 70% of her diet from fats. The BBC reporter advised her not to confuse viewers, and simply say that that everyone should stay away from cakes and biscuits (which is something that we can all agree on). "Missing the point!" I screamed at the telly, "What if the world really isn't flat!"

This tide will turn. The voice of the minority will become mainstream. It has already started to appear in The Body Coach, with some monounsaturated and polyunsaturated fats being called 'healthy fats'. Nutritionists call avocados and nuts 'fit fats'. On the whole we are still too scared to say "eat saturated fat" out loud and proud.

Common sense tells us that our ancestors ate fatty meat, without the risk of heart disease or brain diseases such as dementia. They are modern illnesses that have been created by our modern, processed diets. Heart and brain diseases are created by inflammation.

Cholesterol is a unique and complicated type of fat and it is essential for your body and its functions.

Cholesterol is essential for your body

- Brain synapses are the vital connections between your brain's nerve cells and the rest of your body. They are made almost entirely of cholesterol. Without forming synapses, you can't think properly or remember anything. Your brain needs cholesterol to function as it assists in brain synapses latching the cell membranes together helping to change 'neuroplasticity'. This enables you to become more creative and improves problem-solving. If neurones are useless, they can no longer transmit messages and they die. Dead neurones increase the likelihood of brain disease.

- Low cholesterol levels lead to reduced serotonin levels in your brain. Low serotonin levels are associated with depression. Prozac is a serotonin booster.

- Vitamin D is needed to create healthy bones and to prevent osteoporosis. Vitamin D is synthesised from cholesterol and by sunlight on your skin.

- Cholesterol aids the digestion of fat-soluble vitamins like vitamin A, D and K, so insufficient cholesterol may hinder your ability to digest these vitamins and create an electrolyte imbalance.

- Cell membranes are made from cholesterol. Without it, your cells would disintegrate. Every one of your cells is made up of 50% cholesterol.

- Bile is released from the gall bladder as soon as you eat, helping to digest your food. Cholesterol creates bile acids, which are essential for the absorption of fat from your intestine.

- Cholesterol helps your liver function and clear out toxins like alcohol and medications.

- Cholesterol helps with the production of white blood cells, which are required for prevention of illness and assist the lymphatic system.

- Cholesterol helps the endocrine system communicate with the brain and ensure the efficient, timely release of hormones, including insulin and ghrelin (the 'hunger hormone').

- Cholesterol is a building block for most of your sex hormones, which become particularly important at the menopause..

MYTH-BUSTING SUMMARY

Hormones can't function properly in the absence of cholesterol. The 'hunger hormone' is unable to regulate your appetite and you won't feel satiated.

Cholesterol is essential for brain function

Cholesterol is the fuel for your brain neurones, which rely on the delivery of cholesterol by carrier proteins. Low-density lipoproteins (LDLs) carry cholesterol from the liver to the cells, and high-density lipoproteins (HDLs) carry excess cholesterol back to the liver.

Lipid is the scientific term that encompasses cholesterol, fat and triglycerides. A blood test called a 'lipid profile' measures your total cholesterol (both LDL and HDL) and triglycerides.

- HDLs are often called 'good' cholesterol because they help to stop fat building up in the arteries.

- LDLs are often called 'bad' cholesterol because they lead to fat building up on artery walls.

- Very-low-density lipoproteins (VLDLs) carry triglycerides, another type of fat, to your tissues, and are also deemed 'bad' because they can contribute to the build-up of plaque in your arteries.

High triglyceride levels are an independent risk factor for heart disease. Researchers such as Gary Taubes argue that the triglyceride marker is more important for heart disease risk, because of its associated backbone of glucose. [20] Triglycerides are the hallmark of too many carbs in your diet.[21]

MYTH-BUSTING SUMMARY

LDL, HDL and triglycerides are the fat ratio that you look at when testing for cholesterol. LDL and HDL are proteins and simply *carry* fat molecules. Triglycerides are made up of fat and sugar; when broken down by the body sugar and fats are released. It is the sugar component that scientists are assessing. Therefore, triglycerides are the marker to watch out for in blood tests.

LDL is only an issue when it is 'radicalised'

The problem with LDL is when it gets oxidised. Oxidisation is when a nasty sugar molecule attaches to an innocent LDL protein molecule and changes the molecule's shape. This renders the LDL molecule less useful. 'Less useful'. I love that medical term, 'less useful', which is also known as 'dangerous'. These molecules are dangerous for your body when they hang out with other less desirables and become free radicals.

Free radicals are not harmless, free hippies that have nothing to do. They are a group of subversives who are 'free' to do mischief. Free radicals are proteins that are missing an electron, and what happens when you miss someone? You kick up a storm – in this case a chemical storm. Free radicals are created through any type of oxidative stress. Biochemists call them cells that have become 'biologically rusty'. Oxidative stress comes from daily stress, pollution, chemicals in your toiletries and cleaning products, ultraviolet light, your wheat-based diet and even too much exercise.

Myth-busting summary

LDL is a problem only when it is oxidised.

Free radicals are not innocent hippies; they want to cause mass destruction and create havoc. They start by reducing your resistance to infection, increase your likelihood of getting joint pain and digestive issues. Free radicals increase disorders such as anxiety, headaches, depression and allergies.

Antioxidants, as the name suggests, can impede the oxidation process. Antioxidants can be fat-soluble or water-soluble and free radicals can affect and damage both. Water-soluble antioxidants are easier to access and vitamins E and A and carotenoids are antioxidants (found in vibrantly coloured foods, for instance beta-carotene in carrots) that are fat soluble.

As we age, cholesterol levels naturally increase, as do the free radicals. Cholesterol increases to offer protection against these rampaging free radicals.

TOP TIP

Green tea, berries and vegetables are great sources of antioxidants.

Eat more fat to burn more fat

Simply put, your body can't burn fat if glucose is circulating in your body. I asked a colleague recently, "Why don't people know about this?" and he replied, "Nobody has ever told us." I felt upset that the messages have become confused and adversarial.

Breast milk is 54% saturated fat. Coconut oil is saturated fat. Avocado is monounsaturated fat. Dietary fats do indeed have more calories and your smartphone diet app is going to go off the scale when it reads 'duck' on your macronutrient balance, which is why you are asked to eat lean meat, such as chicken. Apps and dietary guidelines are following the redundant theory that a healthy heart is derived from whole grains. You need dietary fat to assist the function of your heart, head and every cell in your body.

I feel very emotive about the subject of fat. I watched my grannies die very slow and painful deaths. I still remember my dad saying to me when his mum died, "She always listened to her doctor's advice meticulously. Swallowing heart pills and following a low-fat diet all her life. She was starving."

My paternal nan, Eileen, fell over on the bus. The bus driver stopped suddenly and she crashed to the floor, breaking her hip. And so began eight painful years of being unable to stand, sit or even sleep comfortably. A beautiful, gracious lady who was in agony before her death. Living in Wimbledon, my granny and I used to walk up the road to the butchers every day to select the evening meal. Her diet changed, as did so many of ours, the butchers closed, my granddad contracted diabetes.

My nan's low-fat diet meant that osteoporosis afflicted her with heart-wrenching pain for almost a decade. She was a small-limbed, athletic, Irish lady. Small frames have been associated with increased likelihood of osteoporosis. However, my maternal grandmother also had severe osteoporosis and she was tall, with size 7 feet. She was not small-boned.

Low-fat foods featured in Eileen's diet. Agnes suffered with stress, ate a high-carbohydrate diet, and had 'black beneath the eyes' a classic symptom of food intolerances and bad temper. This was undiagnosed at the time: there was rent to pay and mouths to feed. OK, I added the bad temper bit. Without fat in her diet, Eileen was unable to absorb fat-soluble vitamins (A, C and D) or calcium. Her bones were weak, and her demise painful.

Don't calorie count

The diet culture is based on the simple belief that 10g of carbs contains fewer calories than 10g of protein or 10g of fat. Simply, if you eat carbs you are consuming fewer calories. This hypothesis ignores your gorgeous body's chemistry – carbs provide a quick energy burst and you will become hungry again a few hours later. The hunger cycle. Fats and proteins sustain your feeling of fullness and allow you to use 'fatty' deposits in your body to sustain your energy levels for longer.

Going back a step to carbs and insulin, your body has an amazing ability to right itself using insulin. Normal cells are highly sensitive to insulin, which is one of your body's inner guidance systems, but she is exhausted. You can relate to that. The glycaemic index was created to monitor your body's ability to cope with glucose.

An alternative to counting calories is examining your macronutrients. If you are analytical, you can use ratios on your smartphone with apps such as *My Fitness Pal*. I am an intuitive eater and while I used a macro counter in the beginning, I am now happy with a simple formula.

Count 'nutrients' not calories

Counting nutrients is where I spend my time. How many mung beans can I eat in a day? Organic vegetables are expensive, but you are a goddess and you are counting nutrients not calories. Organic veg are high quality and essential for your healthy, gorgeous life.

I have spent thousands of pounds over the course of my life on vitamins and mineral supplements, protein drinks, fizz sticks, reiki massage, shiatsu and massage treatments, but there is no better solution to your health issues than a piece of curly kale. Green veg have so many minerals and vitamins that they are your treasure trove for good health. Eat green veg, every day. Don't count it, measure it, just eat it, lots of it. Eat a whole colour spectrum of veg; count how many different colours of veg you have on every plateful each mealtime. Veg should be part of every meal and snack you have.

Green carbs

Green carbs are veg. You need to eat a lot of veg. Eat as much veg as you can handle on your plate, eat veg as a snack. Pick up a red pepper from your fridge and eat it now. Order an organic veg box to be delivered to your door every week. It is the best thing you can do for your heart, your brain and your body composition (what your body looks like).

Gorgeous Heather hates peas. In fact she hates all vegetables. She said, very emphatically, "Adele, I will work with you, but only if you never make me eat peas." OK I said (with my fingers crossed). Heather was part of a very loving and strict family. Her oldest sister was seven years older and her dad died when she was three. Her mum brought up three kids on a tight budget and was not shy of putting soap in the mouth of a kid who was disrespectful. Painful at the time, but something that Heather said didn't affect her now. It was 'of the time', we agreed.

Respectability and not making a show was a big part of Heather's upbringing. Her mum put a great emphasis on 'keeping up appearances' in front of family and friends. She would often chastise Heather, "It is the exact same place: when you cross the corner of our street you turn into this awful urchin." Heather let go and became difficult as soon as she saw home. Her mum couldn't understand it. Heather had simply had enough of being perfect: who could keep that up? She saw home and relaxed.

Mealtimes were particularly difficult. Heather hated veg, with a passion. She couldn't stand veg. Even as an adult, she would check to see if someone had 'accidentally' put veg on her plate. Her mum never said anything while she was growing up, but the emotion hung heavy. Heather always felt as if everyone was disappointed with her; she was rebellious but the entire act of eating those "slimy, disgusting, vile" veg made her truly sick. She couldn't do it.

If forcing Heather as an adult wasn't going to work, education might. We talked about the nutritious value of veg. Nah! That didn't swing it. So, we talked about why she felt like this – the emotive words that she used describing her veg were fascinating – her words were extremely vivid and rich with expressive emotion.

Heather is a wonderfully caring and nurturing woman, one of the best human resource managers I have ever witnessed in action. We wondered if the expressive Heather had been subdued as a child and veg had become associated with that suppression. Talking about the experiences of mealtimes helped to connect the feeling of lack of control, lack of self-worth and physical pain to... peas. The feelings and tastes are real, but they are associations from childhood. To date, Heather has now eaten 10 peas, but she is far happier with red peppers, which were never on the childhood table – that is a gorgeous result we are still working on.

Eat veg to stabilise your pH

The famous China Study [22] studied the effects of veg on your health and body, naming phytonutrients, the vitamins that you get from veg, as being far superior to meat for your health. This study has been celebrated as the vegan and vegetarian bible for over two decades.

Your amazing body has a pH of 7.4. Do you remember pH from school? The acidity and alkalinity scale? Your body will do whatever it can in many amazing ways, including pulling calcium and magnesium from your bones, to keep your pH of 7.4 stable.

Meat is acid-based. Eating too much meat without vegetables will increase the acidity in your body; vegetables are alkaline and will balance out the pH. Steak and green kale, mung bean and alfalfa salad is a winner. Phew, that is lucky – I know you love a mung bean.

The danger of course is eating too much animal protein without the balancing effect of alkaline veg.

Interestingly, wheat has an even larger acid effect on your body than meat. To make a 'complete protein', you remember that most vegetarians have to use grain and pulse to make a complete protein with the nine essential amino acids in each meal. So refried beans and tacos in Mexico, veggie stew and brown rice, and beans on toast are all examples of complete protein meals that are vegetarian. Just bear in mind that wheat also has a very high acidic load for your body.

Acid reflux, farting and belching may be signs that your husband is home, but they are also signs that his body has too much acid. Ironically, acid reflux is a symptom of too much acid in your diet. More alkaline veg are required.

China Study – bible of the vegetarian diet

A young, vegan, female student was obsessed with *The China Study*. Denise Minger is a statistics whizz, a true academic with a passion for stats. [23] In 2010 she wanted to understand the data and uphold the findings for herself. She was stunned, shocked and dismayed with the reporting. Campbell and Campbell (the authors of *The China Study*) had made a correlation with meat intake without looking at the other variables in the equation; for instance, lifestyle and other dietary habits including consumption of wheat, which also correlated to higher incidence of heart disease.

Fruit and fructose

Janice works as a Neal's Yard consultant. She is highly aware of the nasties in our facial and hair products.

During other discussions she revealed that she was eating a lot of fruit and had tried to use protein shakes with fruit to reduce her weight. She confessed that she had actually gained weight on this route.

Janice's 'healthy' fruit consumption was high, and her reliance on vegetarian shakes was also a cause of concern. She was whizzing up a lot of fruit plus a bit of spinach with her protein shake and eating only that for breakfast, yet she had gained weight.

Fructose is the fruit sugar found in fruits and many other plants. Fructose in an apple is highly watered down when it enters your body; the fibre and the water in the fruit dilutes the fructose sugar. Fruit that is 'processed' in a food blender requires no energy on the part of your body. Your body can assimilate the fructose in a nanosecond. Interestingly fructose has a low glycaemic index. Fructose travels down a very different metabolic pathway from other sugar derivates including sucrose and glucose from bread and sugar.

Fructose isn't digested by your stomach and absorbed by your intestines. Fructose is metabolised almost completely in the liver, in the same way that alcohol is. Fructose and alcohol have the same metabolic pathway through the liver.

If you are consuming a lot of fruit daily, as well as processing a few other pieces of fruit, your liver can't store it all. Your liver can hold only a certain amount. Once it has reached its limit, it sends the rest of the fructose off to storage, in your farthest-to-reach parts of your body: your love handles, tummy, arms, wherever it loves to hang out.

Non-alcoholic fatty liver disease

More importantly, your liver can become saturated if the fructose is coming in fast and your liver can't keep up. Too much fruit leads to non-alcoholic fatty liver disease. Fructose or 'fruit sugar' is found in processed foods like ketchup, yoghurt, soup and salad dressings and it is much more poisonous. Food manufacturers and marketers are very clever at making a product look healthy with images, wording, natural colours and photography to make it look 'clean, healthy, green, fresh'.

Fructose makes you sad

Tryptophan is an amino acid (one of the essential ones you must eat every day) and is essential for serotonin (the happy hormone). Serotonin (a neurotransmitter) connects your brain cells to each other and allows them to chat in a happy and amenable way. The trouble is that fructose binds to tryptophan when it is expelled from the body. No tryptophan = no smiles. Too much fructose can affect your mood.

Serotonin is also an appetite suppressant: it curbs cravings and shuts off appetite. It makes you feel satisfied even if your stomach is not full. The correlation is clear: low serotonin levels mean more cravings.

How much is too much fruit?

Too much fruit is more than three pieces a day. Keep your fruit local. Eat home-grown, indigenous apples and pears. Berries are groovy: blueberries, raspberries, strawberries and pomegranates have a low GI and are high in antioxidants. Processing your fruit in a blender is not a good idea. Eat an apple with cheese and help the digestion to work through your stomach and intestines, leave your liver to work on your occasional glass of wine.

Modern fruit tends to be 'overripe'. Your ancestors ate fruit that was in season and with little ripening; fruit was consumed infrequently and in small quantities.

Beige carbs are basically sugar

Let's get this out of the way. Beige carbohydrates are sugar. Let's not beat about the bush or be apologetic.

QUIZ: Which has the highest GI?

A slice of brown bread, a Snickers bar, a Mars bar, or a banana?

Brown bread.

Here is another – **which has the highest GI?**

White rice, ice cream, cornflakes or white bread?

I bet you got that one right, yes, white bread. Which out of those four has the lowest GI? Ice cream, because of its fat content.

These examples raise two interesting points: first, a slice of white bread is no better for you than a tablespoon of white sugar; second, the GI is a guide, not gospel.

The problem with sugar

Sugar has no nutritional value. Sugar causes diabetes and brain disease. At the beginning of the chapter, I mentioned that carbohydrates are broken down to make glucose.

Glucose and insulin are best buddies; one goes nowhere without the other.

Insulin is seen as the 'darling' or the 'enemy' of the dieter. Insulin is the fat-storing hormone, it mops up the glycogen in your body. Glycogen is a form of glucose broken down from carbohydrates in your body. Your body doesn't care one jot if the carb is from a homemade organic rye slice from Jeff's hippy coffee shop or a piece of millionaire shortbread from the Co-op. It is all sugar to the fanatic. Your body loves it and trips out on it. I'll explain that statement later. Sugar is the only substance in your body that can turn into fat with little effort. Your cells adore sugar, which allows them to hold on to your fat storage.

Body fat must not be squandered by your body at the first sign of physical exercise. Your body is going to hold on to fat because it is valuable and coats all your nerves, makes your brain work and you a 'fast thinker'.

Insulin resistance

Insulin resistance occurs when the cells no longer listen to insulin. Insulin has been shouting at the cells for so long that, like an errant teenager, the cells just tell insulin to shove off. Diabetes and insulin resistance occur when too much glucose is present in the bloodstream, with high levels of insulin, and work by the cells has stopped. Closed for business, too busy, leave us alone, bog off. Every time you eat another banana, cake or slice of bread your body is saturated, overwhelmed and screaming. Your body is quite noisy if you listen to it, rather than the latest fad. The real problem, as discussed earlier, is that 60% of your diet is carbohydrates.

How much is too much carbohydrates?

Great question – I am glad you asked. OK, you have the guidance for fruit and veg, which we answered earlier: three pieces of locally grown fruit and as many kale leaves as you can eat. It is the starchy carbs at every mealtime that is too much. For instance, if you are eating porridge with banana – carbs. Followed by a brown bread sandwich with ham and salad – carbs with a bit of protein. Snack of a Mars bar exclaiming 'everything in moderation', oh the irony. Followed by an evening meal of salmon, brown rice and veg. Carbs, carbs and finally a bit of fat, finished off with a slug of red wine.

Recently I reviewed a low-calorie diet sheet that looked like this:

- Gluten-free oats with pine nuts, almond milk and honey

- Fruit – apple

- Lunch – salad, avocado, ham, low fat cheese, tomatoes, beetroot

- Fruit – either plum, nectarine, strawberries

- Yoghurt – low fat Müllerlight

- Dinner – soup from a tin or home-made soup

- Television time – packet of popcorn

Broadly, this diet contains 99% carbs with high fructose and high-fructose corn syrup and trans-fat in the yoghurt, low-fat cheese and popcorn. There is no break from the glucose spike all day, this is a high-carb, constant-grazing, low-calorie diet. It has very little in the way of proteins and fats.

Some clients understand that food needs to be combined – protein and fat with carbs to lower the GI. But even that doesn't go far enough to satiate your body's needs.

Instead, include eggs and avocado for breakfast (protein and fats). Lunch of cheese salad or tuna salad. Dinner of protein and veg. If you are exercising tomorrow, feel free to add quinoa. Followed off with a slug of camomile tea! "Nice Adele, thanks. But I don't eat…" or perhaps you'll hear yourself say, "I will feel hungry." Have you tried it?

What is wrong with starchy carbs?

Another good question again, I am glad you asked. White carbs are man-made, processed food. There is nothing about them that is natural – no, not even your organic multigrain, wholemeal loaf. We have discussed that there are too many carbs in your diet. The second issue is that they are not natural, they have been man-made, especially wheat. The word 'gluten' is derived from Latin, meaning 'glue'. Glue in modern wheat is what enables Pizza Pete to throw the pizza base around – looks great, but do you really want to eat it? Gluten is also found in hair and body products.

The einkorn wheat that was harvested by Neolithic man was grown as a form of grass seed. Growing and harvesting this grass from the wheat crescent in current day Iran and Iraq (formerly Persia) changed the way people lived and grew. [24]

We became farmers rather than hunters and gatherers and formed the societal, communal relationships that shaped our world as we know it today. Bread remained more or less the same for 2,000 years. At the turn of the last century, scientists began replacing the long wheat with dwarf wheat. Apparently, merging two species of tomatoes to create a hybrid takes no documentation or research. A tomato is a tomato. Wheat is wheat. Einkorn wheat 2,000 years ago had 12 DNA strands, while our wheat has 24. What does the extra DNA do to the consumers? [25]

There has been no research. Scientists simply don't know.

Inflammation causes heart and brain disease

Obsession with dietary fats has meant that we have missed the obvious. *The China Study* had the facts but came to the wrong conclusion. Medical researchers have been systematically reviewing the studies over the past 50 years and uncovered that cholesterol is essential to life and doesn't cause heart attacks. [26]

Malcom Kendrick outlines stress as the cause of inflammation. He asks whether the presence of cholesterol at the site of arterial inflammation indicates that it caused the inflammation or that it is there to heal the inflammation. [27]

Just because cholesterol was holding the smoking gun, did it pull the trigger? Scientists have assumed so. Now other researchers and thinkers are discussing whether dwarf grain wheat pulled the trigger. Dwarf wheat is a toxic chemical that is poison for the body and creates inflammation in your body.

What is a leaky gut?

Leaky gut is created when foreign molecules (like dwarf wheat gluten) have entered the digestive tract and created sore spots and openings into the bloodstream. Alien particles floating around your bloodstream lead to a heightened response from your immune system, which triggers the creation of white blood cells. High alert is raised, and your body creates an overreaction in the form of inflammation. High inflammation for sustained periods of time causes increased cortisol levels and biological stress for your body.

New food items can also enter the blood system through this weakened intestinal wall and create more food allergies that you can throw a stick – or a white blood cell – at. It is called overload.

Immune system triggers and sensitivity to food is caused by leaky gut syndrome. Leaky gut is caused by inflammation. What causes the inflammation?

Toast will give you a buzz

Dwarf wheat's gluten has an ability to bypass the blood-brain barrier. Ideally nothing should get past the brain's defence system. Gluten in dwarf wheat does; gluten is a family of proteins and the composition of gluten is different in the new wheats. You don't want aliens hanging out there, but gluten has managed it and it hits the opiate receptors in your brain. You get high, bread makes you high. You get a buzz from bread, who knew? [28]

The harder it is to give something up, the more you are addicted to it, and that goes for wheat, coffee, chocolate and alcohol. What is your 'deep' reaction to a no-wheat future?

I want you, as a gorgeous girl, to love your treats, but gluten isn't one of them. Researchers suggesting going cold turkey. I have an alternative cunning plan, which I will talk about later.

To resume, the composition of gluten is different in the new wheats and it can pass through the blood-brain barrier, setting in motion the opiate receptors in your brain, which drugs like heroine and morphine also do, without the relief that morphine gives you. Over time this causes inflammation. The interesting thing is your brain doesn't feel pain other than migraines/headaches. The clues are fuzzy head, slight confusion, headaches and migraines. Brain disease is hard to pick up until you have full-blown dementia or Alzheimer's.

Alzheimer's is type 3 diabetes

Research in 1990s revealed the link between Alzheimer's and type 2 diabetes. It showed the direct effect that insulin has to the risk of dementia. Inflammation in the brain leads to brain disease and current thinking is that the brain inflammation – like intestinal and blood inflammation – is caused by the gluten in dwarf wheat. [29]

This feels like another blind alley. You have been here before with cholesterol and dairy produce, but what if it were true? We have been told that heart disease, brain disease, Alzheimer's, cancer and rheumatoid arthritis are all multifactorial. It is a favoured expression – look out for it now I have planted that thought. Cancer is complicated, it is based on many factors. But what if it wasn't? What if the answer has been staring at us in the face for the last 50 years? What has changed over the last 50 years? What makes common sense?

What if Occam's razor, as paraphrased by Isaac Newton, "The simplest case is the most likely," is correct? We have been eating fatty meat for millennia, but we have been eating modern dwarf wheat only for the last 50 years.

The fatter you are, the smaller your brain [30]

Waist and hip measurement has been one of the health principles professionals have worked with for decades. Dividing your waist measurement (above your belly button) by your hip measurement should get you as close to 0.7 as possible. If your waist is more than 35 inches, you are at an increased risk of diabetes. Waist fat, or belly fat, is the sign of visceral fat. Subcutaneous fat sits under your skin and is unsightly but not dangerous. Visceral fat sits on your organs and is dangerous to your organ health and creates more fat because it has more receptors for hormones like cortisol. Cortisol, as we shall discuss later, suppresses the removal of glucose from your body. More of that later, let's move on to what you can do to rebalance and reset your gorgeous body.

Stop drinking probiotic yoghurt drinks

This was the title of one of my highest-ranking blogs. Probiotic yoghurt drinks have very little probiotic and a lot of sugar. Sugar feeds bad bacteria in your gut. Furthermore, you can make your own probiotic drinks and ferment your own or buy foods like kefir and sauerkraut. [31]

Another catchy blog title I have used: **Is your gut flora making you fat?** [32]

Modern humans have about four variants of gut flora. Our ancestor, Neolithic John, had 32 variations of gut flora. To be honest, I don't know exactly how many variations of flora John had, but scientists do know that our ancestors ate 500 different roots and herbs, while our modern diet is derived from just 17 plant crops. [33]

Last summer, while away in France and Spain, everyone in our family contracted a tummy bug. The ferry home from Europe was a 'sticky' affair. We all recovered quickly and went back to school and work on our return. Or did we, did we recover well?

I was bloated and 'overweight' for a long while after and I explained to one of the Gorgeous girls, "My gut flora is making me fat." She laughed, "Yeah, I like that one – it has nothing to do with the patisseries or baguettes." I had increased my intake of carbs while away, but I don't usually gain weight on holiday. My habits are so well embedded and I can get back into the groove when I return and my body keeps me in balance. My gut had been stripped, my defences were low and my weight was increasing.

What makes your gut poorly?

Sickness and antibiotics strip your body of all your bacteria. The natural response to an alien microbe in your body is to get rid of the offending bacteria fast, that is, through sickness and diarrhoea. You remove all good and bad bacteria, which leaves your body defenceless.

However, it isn't just about what you are eating – it can also be caused by stress. Stress can affect your gut because it raises the levels of your stress hormone, cortisol, which can stop your gut from working properly. If you are feeling constant stress, your gut gets rid of food (diarrhoea) so that the energy can go to the brain to deal with the emotional load of stress.

Your immune system is in overdrive and your stomach is very sensitive. Stress inhibits your digestive process and you will be unable to extract the goodness from your food. Most of your serotonin, around 95%, is produced in the cells of your gut; therefore, if your gut is under stress and unhappy you have an unhappy mind, and the cycle continues, leading to your bad health. Eventually everything suffers.

Why do you need good bacteria?

Your gorgeous gut accounts for two-thirds of your immune system and produces 20 hormones; if your gut isn't working properly, you will feel bloated, uncomfortable and unwell.

Good bacteria in your gut will improve your digestion, strengthen your immune system and manufacture the vitamins that your body needs. Bad bacteria will cause digestive problems, mental issues and skin conditions.

Your gut flora can take care of us or it can poison us. 'Chubby bacteria' in your body are attracted to chocolate, cakes and toast. These bacteria are more available because of the lack of diversity of your gut flora. Overproduction of the bad bacteria means that some bacteria can end up in the bloodstream, because of the leaky gut syndrome outlined previously. [34]

In addition, bacteria affect your feelings of satiety and the production of serotonin and dopamine, which come from the amino acids tyrosine and tryptophan. When these 'good' bacteria are fed with probiotics, you stop craving cake and chocolate because chubby bacteria have been starved out.

TOP TIP

Feed your good gut bacteria and starve the bad.

What is a favourite breakfast for good bacteria?

Prebiotics are the food that feeds probiotics. Prebiotics are found in veg like asparagus, leeks and onions. Prebiotics are plant fibres that nourish the good bacteria that already exist in your large intestine.

Probiotics introduce good bacteria into the gut, and prebiotics feed them. Prebiotics act as a fertiliser for the good bacteria. Probiotics are live bacteria and yeasts that are good for your digestive system. Probiotics are beneficial forms of gut bacteria that help stimulate the natural enzymes and processes that keep your digestive organs functioning properly.

When you lose 'good' bacteria in your body (for instance, after sickness or taking antibiotics), probiotics can help replace them. They can help balance your 'good' and 'bad' bacteria to keep your body working as it should.

TOP TIP

When your prebiotics and probiotics work together,
they help your immune system and your mood.

The 'gut-brain connection' affects mood-related disorders, such as anxiety and depression, which are clearly linked to your gut health. Your mood and even your hormonal balance are affected by the state of your body's bacterial inhabitants. [35]

Supplements – do you need them?

You can buy probiotics or you can make your own, for example, kefir. Other supplements, such as protein shakes, are not necessary unless you are doing heavy workouts. Supplements are not a great replacement for real food; the processing required to get the 'protein' from hemp, pea or wheat is so massive that it is no longer digestible by your body.

Any foreign bodies, which are what highly processed foods become, are surrounded by fat and sent to the far reaches of your body (which are scientifically known as love handles or outer thighs). Your body's enzymes and hormones want nothing to do with these foreign bodies. They may claim that they have vitamins XYZ and benefit you with XYZ, but your body hasn't read that label.

When I first started my nutrition journey 20 years ago, I worked with Patrick Holford of Optimum Nutrition and moved through a health continuum. I started with popping vitamins pills like an earnest addict. Open my cabinets and vitamins C and folic acid will fall on top of you. I spent thousands of pounds on vitamins. At 50, I spend nothing on vitamins.

In the fitness industry, I have been offered potions and supplements for decades. Aloe vera, protein powders, metabolism-enhancing supplements. I have tested a wide variety and, apart from fermented foods and organic vinegar, I take nothing now. After decades of being exhausted, running on empty and pushing myself, I now have incredible energy, easily run two businesses, am physically strong with great mental alacrity because I move well, exercise every day, get outside, practise being happy and positive. I enjoy intermittent fasting and carb cycling when I need it. And chocolate!

My body is a fantastic thermostat for my health. If I eat sugary food – cheap chocolate or processed cake – I have an instant headache. Eating a mince pie makes me feel dizzy. I am in tune, I listen, my body tells me instantly.

Being clean means that you can feel the real effects that processed foods have on your body. Please stop putting your head in the sand: your health depends 100% on what you eat. Your productivity at work, and your ability to keep your cool when stress gets too much, comes down to the food you eat. Stop faffing around the edges with different milks, vitamins, alternative therapies and get your 'macros' working for you. Build muscle to support your skeletal frame.

Before leaving this chapter, let's discuss one more trendy cycle of modern nutrition: intermittent fasting (IF). The modern trend of 'grazing' was a culture and a fad I was definitely mixed up in. 'Little and often' was advised to help regulate blood sugar levels. However, we know now that reducing glucose from carbs will regulate insulin and your body can't burn fat with insulin in your body. Intermittent fasting will help your body to clear out its own 'to-do list' and allow your body to have a spring clean. If your amazing body is no longer spending time digesting food, it has time to look after its own jobs.

Does fasting work?

Intermittent fasting is fast becoming – sorry couldn't resist – a big trend in the world of sports and diets. Michael Mosley is a proponent of the 5:2 diet, which indicates the number of days you don't and do fast. Some athletes adopt a 16:8 fasting approach, which indicates the number of hours that you fast – 16 in this case. There are variants, such as 12:12 or 15:9 – the latter simply means that you have 15 hours between your dinner and your breakfast.

I have been using my own version of 12:12 or even 15:9, and have also tried $13^{1}\!/_{4}\!:\!10^{3}\!/_{4}$ intermittent fasting. It has really helped reduce my belly.

While fasting you are keeping good company with Pythagoras and Aristotle, ancient Greeks who felt that purifying their body was akin to purification of the mind. Your mind is sharper and therefore suited to studying. Fasting is also practised in many cultures for spiritual and physical cleansing purposes. It has become one of the most commonplace ways to lose weight; as the pressures of daily life increase, a quick solution is very appealing.

I was very interested in nature's response to fasting and how wounded animals naturally react when they are ill or injured. Serious sickness prompts animals to fast: they are guided by an instinct to limit their intake of food. And of course, all animals adapt themselves to the winter seasons and hibernation. The ability of an animal to fast is nature's best established method of dealing with certain physiological and biological problems.

Hangry fasting

When I first started, my biggest fear was that I would get faint, light-headed and talk rubbish while presenting. In women, fasting can elevate cortisol levels. One of cortisol's effects is that it raises blood sugar. I felt very unsure of fasting and the popular 5:2 diet. I love to exercise, I love the clarity of my mind when I exercise, and I don't want to impede that or feel faint when I exercise and create exercise-induced hypoglycaemia.

Diving into the science of fasting, you learn very quickly the advantages of going without food for a short time. Your body is able to divert energy away from digesting food to cellular repair and the removal of waste material and toxins. This process is called autophagy and it reduces inflammation, enhances biological function and slows down the ageing process. Fasting also speeds up a process called apoptosis whereby your body rids itself of old, unhealthy cells and replaces them with new ones.

Human growth hormone (HGH) increases by as much as five times during intermittent fasting. The higher your levels of HGH, the easier it is to burn fat and maintain your muscles. [36]

Intermittent fasting will result in a considerable effect on fat loss because of the decrease in insulin and the corresponding increase in nor-epinephrine (or nor-adrenaline in UK) – the main neurotransmitter produced by the sympathetic nervous system. This cocktail of hormones initiates the breakdown of stored body fat and uses it as an energy source.

Plus, the big win is that research indicates that a large percentage of the weight lost from intermittent fasting comes from stored belly fat. It also helps with anti-ageing because of the increased production of the HGH, which stimulates the growth of new cells and smoother skin – OK, I added the smoother skin. I would rather fast than add chemical creams. [37]

Some studies demonstrate that intermittent fasting can increase the growth of new neurones and increase brain function. Neuroplasticity and increased cognitive function raises levels of a brain hormone called brain-derived neurotrophic factor (BDNF), a deficiency of which is associated with higher rates of depression, learning difficulties and memory loss. [38]

Warning: women, fasting and increased cortisol

Fasting is an absolutely different thing from starvation. One is beneficial, the other harmful. One is valuable and is a therapeutic measure based on resting your digestive process for a while and allows the body to adjust and adapt, allowing your body to heal.

Some evidence suggests that intermittent fasting is not as beneficial for women: it may worsen your control of blood sugar level. Personally, I believe this may be down to your body type. If you are an ectomorph (with a lean and delicate build of body, like Gwyneth Paltrow, Kate Moss, Cameron Diaz) who can tolerate a lot of carbs, in fact need carbs and therefore glucose to feel energised, you are going to struggle with an intermittent fasting schedule. Your body works better with carbs, which means that you are burning a lot of sugar, so if that body type starts to burn glucose, they are going to become dizzy and disorientated and hangry.

If, like me, you are more of a mesomorph (with a compact and muscular build, like Halle Berry, Madonna and Jessica Alba) then an intermittent fasting routine is more likely to work for you. This applies also to endomorphs (who have a soft, round build of body and a high proportion of fat tissue, like Kim Kardashian, Beyoncé and Jennifer Lopez).

Intermittent fasting and being hangry

Making sure your diet is on track first is essential. If you are eating cereal, toast, sandwiches and evening meal pasta, you are on a high-sugar diet and you will go into sugar withdrawal and perhaps hypoglycaemia. When you are burning glucose like this, you are going to become 'hangry'. The insight or the trick is to get a good diet with minimal sugars and reduced carbs before starting intermittent fasting. Then when you move into an intermittent fasting routine you will start to burn fats and produce ketones, which is fat burning in ketosis. I will talk about this and its link to exercise in the last chapter. For now, get your macros right and then start intermittent fasting by noticing how long you go from dinner to breakfast and simply making that time longer and longer.

TOP TIP

Try intermittent fasting, carb cycling,
fresh air and good movement.

"Can you help me with rheumatoid arthritis, fibromyalgia, heartburn, or anxiety?" These are the wrong questions to ask. These issues can be solved with lifestyle changes: there is no pill. You simply need to stop fretting about the latest food fad, be open-minded and more flexible in your thinking and listen to your body. Begin simply to reduce your intake of carbs and eat more fat and protein. Enjoy life. And eat more veg – obviously!

"You may very well say that, Adele, but eating veg (or exercising or eating meat or fewer carbs or finding the time or my unhelpful husband) is a real problem for me."

"I am sure it is, Gertrude, but I am really concerned that your health is suffering, very badly, and you need to get out of your own way."

Your current health issues can be sorted. You can have a fantastic little waist and great energy, be free from mental anguish, and rid yourself of diets and portion control, but you have to do the groundwork. You have to set your vision and follow your path.

CHAPTER 7

Health starts with your mental health

Stress is widely written about, talked about, worried about. It is of course linked to your health and – perhaps less well known – your weight.

Cortisol belly

'Cortisol belly' doesn't roll off the tongue as well as 'meno belly' or 'wheat belly', but cortisol belly is a thing, apologies, a scientific thing. [1]

Cortisol raises blood sugar because it shuts off insulin. Cortisol is the 'stranger danger' hormone that moves you into a sense of high alert. Getting ready to run, to avoid your attacker or stand frozen to the spot in fear, or ready with your handbag to take a swing (or maybe if you are a modern woman it's a taser gun – that is illegal, and I've been watching too many Swedish films). The point is you are terrified, on high alert and your body is waiting to respond. Whichever way you choose to go, you need energy and you need swift, alert responses quickly.

Cortisol wants you to have the capability to react to danger; it wants you to be able to run across the road, or lift a heavy piece of wood all to save Freddy from a car or falling tree. You have superhuman, lightning-speed reactions because cortisol makes glucose readily available in your bloodstream, so you can go, go, go. Insulin is switched off and therefore unable to shuttle the glucose into fat or muscle storage. The glucose is left in your bloodstream as long as cortisol deems it necessary – 'Queen Cortisol' has the power.

But what if it wasn't a falling tree or near-death experience for Freddy? What if it is an annoying neighbour, or a car that doesn't start, or a boss or co-worker that you kindly want to smack? Whether you smack him or not, you still have the emotional and physical debris of the encounter. Cortisol, or 'Queen Cortisol' as I like to describe her, won't be leaving the building until she is good and ready.

High periods of stress can increase your blood sugar and allow glucose to be readily available to your muscles, so that you can run or punch. There is no insulin to remove it. After prolonged periods of time with high glucose, when insulin is finally allowed in, it has a massive job and your pancreas can't produce enough insulin, but it keeps going. Your cells get fed up with all the shouting and insulin-ting (just created a new word for insulting insulin) and reacts like a teenager. You have heard this story before with diabetes and glucose and insulin, but this time it's cortisol that is creating the same toxic environment in your body.

Among all the screaming and shouting, your cells still don't get any energy, because the sugar is in the bloodstream and not being transported effectively to where it needs to be.

It is similar to when you and your partner argue over who is going to feed the cat and, in the end, the poor cat doesn't get fed at all. If your cells don't get fed, then like the hungry cat meowing for food, they send out hormone signals for more food (OK, I am going to walk away from the cat analogy).

Thus your appetite is stimulated, which means you reach out for comfort food: sugars and trans-fats (I won't refer to high fat, only trans-fats, let's be clear) like cakes, doughnuts, chocolates and so forth, and who wouldn't? You reach for comfort food when you are stressed. Your cells want glucose; even though it is in your body already, it is not where it needs to be.

Cortisol increases your heart rate, pumps more blood and gets your body ready for quick action, for which it needs a lot of energy. Cortisol inhibits insulin production to prevent glucose from being stored, so that it can be used immediately. But you don't run or do any physical exercise, so cortisol mobilises triglycerides (remember them: fat with glycerol backbone; glycerol also known as sugar) from storage and relocates them to visceral fat in the belly.

Visceral fat, as we discussed earlier, is belly fat. It surrounds your organs and is the worst type of fat. Subcutaneous fat simply hangs off your arms and hips and isn't so bad (says who!). Visceral fat has more cortisol receptors than subcutaneous fat. Cortisol sits on your belly, hence the term 'cortisol belly'.

Cortisol is a catabolic hormone: it breaks down muscle. You see hyperactive, nervous personality types who are skinny, with no muscle – this is due to high cortisol levels. Muscle is needed to help with the ageing process and keep your joints happy for great posture.

TOP TIP

So, the easy answer is:
don't eat wheat and don't ever get stressed!

That may be just a little easier said than done, and you have probably just called me a facetious so and so. I would suggest that awareness is your best defence. Being knowledgeable and aware of your own biochemistry and taking a moment to consider the effect of stress on your body will give your inner goddess the upper hand. It will give you a few seconds to quieten down Horace or Rose, your inner stress critic. In my opinion, knowledge is also a habit interruption strategy.

What is a meno belly?

During menopause, the 'meno belly' becomes more evident. The question is why at the menopause? It is all to do with another part of your endocrine system (hormones). Again, this time it isn't insulin.

When you reach the menopause, your gorgeous body stops using your ovaries to secrete the sex hormones, including oestrogen and progesterone. Your 28-day cycle is governed by the rise of oestrogen at the beginning of your cycle, egg released and testosterone brings your oestrogen back down. Amanda Hamilton in her book *Eat, Fast, Slim* outlines the menstrual cycle in beautiful, simplistic detail if you are interested in finding out more. [2]

Balancing your hormones is essential throughout your life, but in particular during your menopause, because our bodies have become more oestrogen-dominant due to the excessive oestrogen that we are exposed to in the food cycle and in the products we use.

Oestrogen dominance

Why? Hormones are in our water system, thanks to flushed contraceptive pills. [3] There are added hormones in chicken, and cattle feed. Soya (or soy) is another issue. Soya that is fermented, like miso or tempeh, is good for your digestion and includes vitamin K2, which is needed for your nerve health, muscles and bones.

However, the issue with soya products, such as tofu, soy protein isolates (found in protein shakes and protein bars), soya milk, soya flour and in many processed foods is that they are full of phytoestrogens called isoflavones that mimic oestrogen in your body.

For these reasons, you may be oestrogen-dominant, especially if you are a vegetarian eating a lot of unfermented soya. Don't freak out: simply eat fermented soya.

At the menopause this all becomes even more important when oestrogen and testosterone start to become further imbalanced and decline. Mix in increased cortisol due to high stress levels and menopause symptoms become screamingly good fun. If you are interested in finding out more, head over to my YouTube channel and also listen to Dr Berg's explanation of oestrogen, mood and menopause. [4,5]

Women have reduced risk of heart disease – why?

Women create a problem for the cholesterol hypothesis or lipid debate. It has been widely recognised for many years that women generally suffer much less heart disease than men – especially younger, premenopausal women. The difference is usually 300%, yet woman have higher average cholesterol levels. [6]

This created the theory that women are protected from raised cholesterol levels by their sex hormones, which would accord with the protection disappearing after the menopause. This theory has been proved to be incorrect.

In a 1963 study, two groups of women who had undergone gynaecology surgery were compared. The first group were producing no hormones: their ovaries had been removed. The second group had had hysterectomies, but their ovaries were intact, and some hormones were still being produced. The findings concluded that there was no difference between the incidence of coronary heart disease in the two groups. Therefore, it was not hormones or ovary function that is responsible for the fact that women suffer from fewer heart attacks. [7]

"It was never the female sex hormone. Instead it is the fact that women generally have higher HDL levels and this protects against heart disease."

Dr Malcom Kendrick [8]

The idea that the female sex hormone protected against heart disease came into existence to provide an explanation for the alleged female 'protection' against raised cholesterol levels. It is an example of scientists jumping to a scientific yet flawed conclusion.

The real reason for a menopause belly

A stress belly is created after the menopause because your ovaries go into natural decline. This is absolutely groovy and fine, as they have done an amazing job, and it's time for them to retire and allow other organs to take over the production of progesterone and oestrogen. Production of these essential hormones falls to the adrenal glands, which are situated above your kidneys.

On a scale of 1 to 10, how 'fit' and ready are your adrenal glands to take on another job? What have your stress levels been like in the first 50 years of your life? Calm and peaceful, with lots of trips to Indian yoga retreats and health farms, no alcohol and no inflammation to deal with? Do you have low cortisol levels? No, thought not, who does? Well, during the menopause your adrenal glands have another job, which is producing and balancing low level sex hormones.

If the above did happen and your adrenal glands are happy to take on one more job, then your hormone levels at the menopause will return to the levels they were before adolescence. Your hormones will return to where they were as a kid. That wouldn't be a problem.

But if your adrenal glands have been pumping cortisol into your body for the last 50 years as you feed the cat, answer emails, put on make-up and eat cereal, they aren't going to be fit enough for another job. Decreasing your stress levels and creating a calm mindset is going to help your menopause symptoms. Habit interruption strategies are a great way to release stress, but let's talk about that later.

Your meno belly is caused by stress

Dr Malcom Kendrick systematically reviewed the countries where the incidence of heart attacks had increased the most over the previous five decades. Forced removal from your home and the destruction of your community is the biggest 'stress' load a human can feel. Imagine: no friends, no home, no social connections, upheaval and ties broken. Forced displacements have been associated with an increased incidence of heart attacks. For instance, Finland was forcibly repatriated into Russia in the 1970s and had the largest blip in heart disease. [9] In the 1980s, when Communism began to lose its grip, the Berlin Wall came down, and the entire Soviet bloc was plunged into chaos; this affected the health of the eastern Europeans for the following decade.

Glasgow, with it is culinarily delights of deep fried Mars bars, had a history of demolishing its slum areas, including the Gorbals, and displacing families to the outlying areas of Cumbernauld and elsewhere. And yet bigger cultural changes have affected the health of entire populations. The Australian Aboriginals have seen their culture, lifestyle, status and communities completely shredded. Maoris in New Zealand and Native Americans in USA and Canada have the worst health indicators in the world.

Migration is another key indicator of heart issues, especially among the Indian emigrants to predominantly Christian countries such as the UK, USA or Australia; a cultural change that can feel stressful for the first generation of migrants. These displacement changes showed a correlation to high levels of stress and high levels of heart disease. [10]

Whether this theory stands the test of time remains to be seen and rigorous research is under review; however, the fact-finding data illustrates that stress needs to be taken very seriously.

Be stress aware

Awareness and knowledge are your first defence in managing stress and avoiding unhealthy visceral belly fat. Even if your inner diva wants to let rip, hold on a second and listen to the consequences that will have on your tummy and more importantly your life in general. Ask Julie the diva to sit quiet.

Stress can be created in a number of ways, from worrying about what people think of you, to repetitive thoughts that simply won't go away, or what train you are going to catch on Thursday next week to get to a meeting on time. It is all very well for self-proclaimed expert and psychoanalyst 'hubby' to say, "Well don't worry about it, let it happen and unfold." That simply puts the stress register up a notch further. Few empathy points lost there, master guru of nothing. The point is it is stressful for you.

Being irritable with loved ones and not getting enough sleep to be rationale because you are stressed about the train, rain or dog is all part of the mix. The answer lies with you; it always does. Ask yourself, "How can I best deal with this?" Use a simple statement to find the solution in your brain: it will give you a moment, break the repetitive thought and give your goddess an opening. That is all she needs. Your higher self, your neocortex, your brain will find a happy path.

Your emotions influence your body's chemistry

Biochemistry tells us that our hormone levels are influenced by our emotions – the last section proved and outlined that very clearly. The wonderful, positive thing is that doesn't go one way. I appreciate that you may feel that you have been hijacked by your emotions and you can't climb down from the Queen Cortisol throne, but you can, and it is very easy.

Your biochemistry can also work for you. You can harness your biochemistry to create a calm space. Use your own biochemistry to stimulate your senses, create a peaceful aura and improve your circulation and aid cellular repair. Before you roll your eyes and think this means going up a Himalayan mountain to gather pink sea salt and sit with an Indian yoga guru clad in a loincloth, in a dark cave, just alert your senses to the feeling of calm that humour can engender.

Let me give you a quick insight into our family and marital background. I was raised in a Scottish Catholic background with a bit of Irish maverick hippy madness thrown in. It means I am not good with swearing: it is a sin, a cardinal sin. I do it, but it makes my toes curl. When the situation gets tense in our family environment, when my hubby Dave has left the milk out once too often or forgotten to put his shoes away again – yes, I am talking high stress – and the situation has exploded because I am busy or tired or hangry or stressed and I quite rightly give him a right royal rollickin', the mood is edgy. Which way will the next few hours go? Dave swears! I mean, he really lets rip and swears very badly. I scream with laughter. I can't believe what I am hearing; it is hilarious. My energy has instantly transformed into shock and then unbelievable hilarity. You'd think after 20 years that it would lose its impact, but no, it still works every time.

You can shift your emotions

First you need to notice them, feel your emotions. I ask clients this all the time and sometimes a client will understand me instantly. Where do you feel that pain in your body? I loved working with Abigail from Cornwall because she could feel it instantly; she used to tell me that her pain was a football, a massive football in the centre of her belly. She was stuffing the football down her throat all the time. Her trigger was seeing kids' pain, kids who were suffering because of a bad marriage or ill treatment because of a stressed adult. Any curious female is going to know where that has come from. The point is that the football was an emotional block and it wasn't being attended to: the pain was being stuffed back down with cream cakes.

Do you keep your stress in your belly?

Your emotional awareness may involve a delicate stomach. Do you keep your stress in your belly; does your belly twitch and quiver? Or does it react badly to certain foods? Your gut, as explained in the last chapter, is your second brain and is where you feel your 'gut instinct'. It may well be a foreign object entering your bloodstream, as described by the term 'leaky gut', but it is also an emotional indicator. Tightness in your stomach is the clue to how you are feeling.

It doesn't have to be your tummy it could be your heart, a heart pain, not a chest clenching heart attack feeling but simply an ache or an emptiness. Fiona had completely dissociated herself from her body. She had been overweight since her university days and found attaching her thoughts to her body very difficult. We started with her pretty toes, how beautiful her toes were, admiring her toes, painting the nails and massaging them. In time, she moved up to realise she had beautiful ankles, really feminine. Over the weeks she recognised how much she liked her shapely calves. How strong and athletic they looked, and she began accepting her body one small step at a time.

Start noticing your pretty toes and manage your stress. Please don't suppress your footballs by hating your body. I heard a client call her body "the thing that transports me, it gets me around. I clothe it, feed it and move on." What pain, what misery; why would you look after something that made you feel like that?

Notice where your emotions sit in your body

Respect your symptoms – I have a pain in my heart, a dullness in my thoughts, a despair in the pit of my stomach – and reclaim them. Look into the pain and acknowledge it. Knowledge can help your habit interruptions strategy. Why do I feel like that? You may never get to the bottom of why the pain is there exactly; remember those *in utero* conversations from earlier? Your emotional memory may have been set before you were born or before you had a real knowledge of the world, and you were simply acting upon the emotion of the event, rather than the facts. In my humble opinion, there is no need to go back and uncover all past hurts; simply acknowledge them. Recognise that an emotion is there and what your misdiagnosed mindset is telling you and what these thoughts are teaching you about yourself.

Gorgeous Claire's stress was caused by holding together a very busy job as a solicitor and her life with two boy screenagers and a sad hubby. Barry had a negative mindset about life, and had 'proper' issues, according to Claire. It meant that she couldn't look after herself; she didn't have time because she was dealing with his moods and life reactions. She was living on eggshells, and her stress levels were high. Claire and I worked through how she could remove these obstacles. I could see her gold; I knew her goddess would work through the answers. She had the key. She explained that Barry had tried psychotherapy, but had been told that his issues were so awful that it would take "thousands of pounds and three years to uncover" so he decided against it. Claire was dealing with somebody's else's mindset block, unfortunately. Working around that can prove difficult.

Coaching involves action, asking the tricky questions and uncovering the truth and the emotion behind the action or thought. But here is the rub: you can listen to yourself and coach yourself. You can be self-aware. Reclaim your own journey, acknowledge your feelings rather than suppressing them and know that headaches, stomach aches and little toe pain are clues, insights. Welcome your stress and your shouting matches: they are little bombshells of insights. How curious! Remember Zander, the conductor?

Insight bombshells

Go back to biochemistry if your body is feeling overwhelmed, your mind frazzled, you are just about to deal with a high-alert situation like leaving early from work to get to an appointment across town. You know life and death situations like Bruce Willis's towering inferno scenarios. How to deal with the situation once you are aware of it?

Recall your special time

Before you rush off, find some space and recall a time in your life when you experienced total pleasure. It may be that you walk outside to clear your thoughts and lift your spirits. For instance, Dave and I climbed Ben Nevis a few years ago in April. We parked our 'van with a bed' motorhome overnight and were ready to jump out and climb early in the morning. The summit was heaven. It was one of the three days that Scotland has sunshine – sorry, typo, when Ben Nevis has sunshine – and it was glorious. The weather was incredible, I was physically knackered, which is always a personal high and it was a gift. Open, fresh and uninhabited – it was amazing. What is your memory; what is it that makes you feel calm and lifts your heart?

Repeat your personal mantra

The personal mantra, "I love myself" works. Say it. Chant it, sing it, tell your colleagues. Raise your vibration. What is your personal affirmation? My stress workshops always sell out quickly, as there is clearly a need for them. Beforehand, I ask attendees to think of their most memorable place in detail, so we can go there in our meditation, and also to think of a mantra that I refer to again in the meditation. I also offer a few of my own affirmations to keep the atmosphere calm and peaceful.

On one occasion, I was practising my mindful, guided meditation, relaxing and chillaxing and letting go of the day's worries. Within the room, the doors were open to the garden and a light breeze moved gently through the room. The day was comfortably warm and the guests all had blankets and were snoozing lightly – or meditating deeply. With my eyes closed, in my own world, describing how the guests' bodies may feel and letting go and dropping deep, I asked the group to let go of their worries and begin to feel the energy of their memorable place and affirm their own personal mantra.

Scratch the record player, noise, disruption, confusion from the back of the room, as an anguished guest couldn't remember her mantra. It was a long, carefully considered paragraph. She didn't want to miss anything. So, she got up, stepped on someone's glasses and found her mantra. I would lovingly suggest that your mantra is easy to remember.

Being mindful not mind full

Using the tips of awareness: knowledge is power, and insights are clues, you have the strategy to know yourself and the tactics to help you to stop your normal routine and behaviour. You can use a simple habit interruption strategy of asking yourself a pertinent question, and coach yourself through the stressful situation. This will change your focus and allow you to become more present and more mindful. Voicing out loud, writing and journaling how you are feeling will give you a powerful insight into your own thinking.

Once you can see, hear, and feel your blocks, you can use techniques to stop your adopted behaviour and decide if you want to create a new neural pathway, a new direction in your life without stress. For instance, Pilates, tai chi and yoga are all mind-body techniques and offer you a physical insight into the way your body moves and perhaps even an emotional release as well. Many times, clients have cried in Pilates or my meditation practice. Letting go is an essential part of your health; releasing suppressed emotions frees your body from physical and emotional pain.

Mindful techniques

Other simple mindful techniques include being present as you place a plate down on the table, eating slowly and noticing the colours and the textures of the food. Walking very slowly and reciting your personal mantra is a great habit to cultivate.

Music is also a personal love. Floating, ethereal music – whether classical music or chanting dolphins – I am interested. I rebelled against classical music as a kid, but as a new mum I used it as a tool to sedate gangster toddlers; having it in the background as they were playing had an amazing effect. Teaching Pilates is a dream with the right ambience and music – and of course amazing clients.

Easy rituals that you create can help calm your thoughts throughout your day as well as being actions to take in high-stress situations. Rituals that allow you space to think what you want from your day. In *Memoirs of a Geisha*, the author outlines the first role of a geisha: to practise the art form of making tea. It was a very powerful practice that allowed emotions to be heightened. Physical, unspoken language becomes more expressive and small gestures become magnified.

Working with this awareness tool, make simple, mindful habits a part of your natural day. This will enable you to make a difference to how you cope with sudden stress, and the increased awareness in your day will create even more insights.

Gorgeous Lisa, a retail director manager for a huge multinational company, wanted to work on her health and wellbeing and lose a few pounds. She works abroad; her job requires a lot of travel. She knew that "something had to give." Working long hours, she was constantly exhausted. She had a few physical issues from an injury that needed attention, and she wanted to get back to full fitness. Part of Lisa's rehab was physical. She needed to train her quads and fire off her glutes a little more and stretch her deep-seated piriformis muscle. Easy biomechanical stuff, which over time we healed together.

Work was a side issue that kept popping into the conversation as a barrier. When I suggested that she didn't go down to dinner with her male colleagues and instead spent some time on using our videos to strengthen her core and increase her musculature to support her frame, work kept getting in the way. She explained, "When I am at work, I work. I can't leave my colleagues. They need me to be there. Look, I just need to get through the next seven years, then I will have accumulated enough funds and time in this job, and I can move on and begin my life."

What an insight; what an interesting statement. The penny dropped almost as soon as she spoke the words. "I am in survival mode, I can't live like this, I want to enjoy my life now." As soon as the revelation appeared, other mindset setbacks came down in quick succession.

Alcohol also played a big part in Lisa's role. Her male colleagues, away from home, drank a lot and she didn't want to miss out on the important conversation and deals that were brokered at the bar. As a woman, she didn't want to be different or to miss out on decisions that would affect the business. She felt she needed to be a part of the negotiations, whereas in reality it was a lack of confidence that was the issue.

Lisa began to realise that the important conversations were not happening in the bar. Her boss used to ring her after the drunk evenings, to establish what had been agreed and obtain her thoughts. Her boss was contacting her, her advice was being sought. She wasn't missing out, out of the loop: she was the loop. Lisa stopped joining her colleagues in the bar and felt safe in her room, knowing that the meeting would come to her.

Eating was another issue. Colleagues wanted to eat takeaways, and she might appear weak if seen to be on a diet. Then Lisa realised she was not on a diet: she was creating better eating habits and living a healthy lifestyle so that in the morning she could broker a better deal for her company. She was in control and had the jurisdiction to move the company debate forward; she held the power strings and needed to be clear-headed in order to do that. Lisa was making decisions for her health that supported optimum performance at work. That simple reframe freed Lisa from the 'diet' mindset. Her male colleagues may well have been derisory about a weight loss plan, but not about a "with a clear head, I am about to outperform you – you'd better get your act together" plan.

Practise self-care

Allocating time for yourself and time for relaxation is anathema to most women. I post a self-care Sunday practice on Instagram each week to make the habit stick.

Include some 'free' practices, such as baths, walks, nature, painting your toenails, reading a light novel. Other inexpensive practices can include candles, luxury chocolates, dimmed lights, buying yourself flowers. I love flowers. I started buying daffodils and worked up. I love daffodils – they are yellow, happy and resilient. I upgraded and worked through my financial 'spending-money-on-myself' hang-ups.

Practise your self-care every day. Give yourself an emotional break from your inner critic and be kind to yourself. If your boss or family member is giving you a hard time, talk to them, open up and see where that leads. Don't play their game; don't increase the stress stakes. Step back and look for a way round. You are gifted with the resources to do that.

Adrenal fatigue is real

Menopause fatigue and burnt-out adrenals will make your menopause symptoms worse. Constantly using your survival gland to fight, flight or freeze will exhaust you. Constantly solving problems in your head is a sign of adrenal fatigue, as is the frustration that can arise when faced with seemingly incompetent or slow people. The symptoms of adrenal fatigue are brain fog, hair loss and fluid retention.

As you are probably aware, I am in awe of your amazing body and its ability to heal and regenerate. Your cells regenerate all the time, and we've discussed your brain's ability to learn new pathways, known as neuroplasticity.

Your body heals itself via your nervous system.

Your autonomic nervous system has two balancing components: the survival mechanism of the sympathetic nervous system; and its opposite, the parasympathetic nervous system, which allows you to rest and digest, and releases the body's energy to heal on a subconscious level. Your body can reset and will do that on your behalf, but it needs your attention and time to do that.

Enhance your 'rest and digest'

Concentrating on your breath as you move around your office will improve the function of your pituitary gland, located in your brain, which secretes hormones that can naturally subdue and sedate your Cortisol Queen.

To start the day right, make a conscious effort to get up as soon as you hear your morning alarm. Don't hit the 'slumber' or 'snooze' buttons. Get up before your brain conducts an inner dialogue explaining that you are warm and cosy. Get up. Set a routine and this habit will become fixed. I reset my disrupted hormonal sleep pattern by setting my alarm for 6am every morning. This means that after years of having an overactive, can't-sleep brain at night, I now go to sleep instantly and wake up before the alarm, and go over my gratitudes. It is a gift and a habit that I will no longer surrender. The gift of a full night's sleep is important to me, way more than a few extra minutes, 10 annoying minutes during which I talk to my inner critic at length. I leave Angela (my inner critic) in bed and get up to enjoy a morning of doing what I want to do. The first thing is to fix my hubby a cup of tea and me a glass of hot water with lemon, and to do a few foot stretches while there. Then I can relax and enjoy waking up.

If you are getting up late, consuming coffee and shoving cereal down your throat, answering emails, planning pick-ups and drop-offs with hubby, listening to the news (or worse, Radio 1), making sandwiches for the family and trying to apply make-up, that is how your whole day will continue. Set your intention for the day. Start your day well and create a calm intention for the rest of your day.

Valuing yourself is countercultural

As women, we value our friends, our kids, our workplaces, our communities, our cats, our dogs, even our next-door neighbours' cats. Everybody and everything gets 'fed' before us – metaphorically and physically. Why do you have to do everything? What does it say about you that you are the only one that can handle all these jobs?

A big part of my stress workshop is forgiveness. Over the years, I have had various responses: hurt, upset and anger. Forgiveness is hard for some people, understandably. Forgiving a transgressor can be extremely painful, especially if that transgression occurred to an innocent person. Watching or being part of cruelty and being unable to help or defend yourself is indescribably painful and that situation is unforgivable. Holding that pain means that you are drinking poison every day: drinking poison, hurting yourself and expecting that horrible person to drink the poison. You are hurting yourself more by reliving the experience or holding a grudge against that individual. Letting go is a state of mind: it takes practice, but you can heal yourself.

Feeling your emotions is an imperative part of healing. Feeling into your intuition will guide you forward. Taking your time to do this is a habit to cultivate, honour and respect as much as you respect and love yourself.

Lack of sleep is a big weight gainer. If you are not sleeping well because of shift work or stress, you are likely to gain weight. Maintaining a self-care sleep routine is important for your wellbeing. Keep all electronic equipment out of your bedroom: no blue lights from electronics or clocks. Your brain is designed to wake up from a blue light, so keep things subdued and the lights low.

Is your bedroom a storage space or a love nest? Which environment will aid better sleep? Spend the time in your bedroom only for sleep and dressing. Your body will understand the message. Circadian rhythms are essential to restful sleep, so get up and go to bed at the same time every day, including weekends. You can't outrun a bad diet and you can't catch up on bad sleep from the week. Get up and sleep deeply the next night.

CHAPTER 8

Good health includes everyday movement

How do you feel when you have finished a class of Pilates, or a swim, or a cycling session? Fulfilled and happy? Regular exercise and, more important, daily movement will improve your sleep, increase your overall energy and your self-confidence, decrease your stress levels and reduce your risk of illness.

Being active will help to reduce inflammation and cleanse your system, which will reduce your risk of heart disease and diabetes by increasing your sensitivity to insulin, which helps to control your blood sugar levels.

Being physically active will reduce your risk of osteoporosis. Brittle bone disease can be extremely painful and normally occurs later on in life. Bone mass continues to grow until the age of around 30, and is maximised by regular exercise. The more exercise you do, the greater your peak bone mass tends to be. After the age of 30, bone mass starts to deteriorate unless you carry on exercising.

Your 'body composition' refers to the ratio of lean tissue to fat, the ratio of muscle and organs to your fat distribution. If you are carrying excess fat, it is detrimental to your health, because of the strain on your joints and your organs.

What type of exercise?

General recommendations are for activity five times a week, getting out of breath for about 30 minutes. Ideally, however, you should be aiming for much more movement than this: 10,000 steps a day plus 30 minutes' exercise five days a week across three varied discipline platforms: cardiovascular, strength and postural.

Cardio exercise is for your heart and lungs. *Strength training* is for your bones and increased muscle power. A *body-mind discipline*, such as yoga, Pilates or tai chi helps to release your myofascia and your ability to stretch, so that you can perform other activities in your daily life.

Cardio exercises, which include activities such as running, power walking and swimming, should make you 'out of breath' and help maintain your respiratory and heart function. Aerobic exercise turns on your longevity genes and your brain's 'growth hormone' and reduces memory decline. There is an extraordinary relationship between physical fitness and mental fitness. [1]

Weight and strength training are essential for bone health and body composition. Research into muscle strengthening and resistance training has shown that it helps to prevent rapid aging. A review found that progressive and sustained resistance exercise will improve not only muscle strength, but also your walking speed and gait. It improves your overall physical ability and corrects any functional limitations so that you can move and use your limbs effectively and with ease. [2]

Weight-bearing exercise for the prevention of osteoporosis

Given my grandmothers' experiences, osteoporosis is a concern for me, especially with my body frame. I have small bones (not bottom) and a slight frame, which means bone density is at risk. I have less bone to lose than women with larger frames. This is one of the reasons I won't dabble in removing milk and dairy from my diet. Of course, you can obtain calcium from dark green, leafy vegetables – broccoli, kale, cabbage and watercress. Dried fruits, nuts, seeds and pulses (peas, beans and lentils) are all excellent sources of calcium. I eat all of these, but full-fat milk and cheese are also staying in my diet.

TOP TIP

Don't forget about vitamin D, which enables your body to absorb calcium, and is found in egg yolks, oily fish (including salmon, sardines and tuna) and wild mushrooms.

As mentioned earlier, weight-bearing exercise is essential for bone health, but bad posture can affect your bone density. If you are constantly stooping forward, your gorgeous body will notice that your back doesn't have any forces to deal with and therefore stop providing bone formations to your shoulders and upper back. Your bad posture will start to have a negative and degenerative effect on your bone density over time. Your body is efficient: it won't work or use energy if you are not using it. If you are not upright, if your shoulders are not in line with your body, and if your upper back is rounded, your body will efficiently decline to add any bone density. Great posture is essential for your bone health. Sitting in the same posture for hours, weeks and years will have a detrimental effect on your physiology, but also zaps your body of energy.

TOP TIP

Create good posture while sitting,
standing and walking.

In the exact way that your emotions are the key to your emotional health, your aches and pains are clues to your physical health. A slightly annoying, recurring headache or foot pain is your body talking to you. Your body, once heard, is very noisy and a mind-body discipline will get you closer to hearing and noticing what your body is saying.

The term 'functional training' has been used in the fitness industry for quite some time. The exercises used in functional training focus on the muscle groups that help you function in your everyday life.

Remedial exercise such as Pilates is vital for your health. Pilates is a form of functional exercise that improves your ability to move quickly, turn abruptly, swivel or twist at a moment's notice. Practising these functional moves in a class and every day could help make your entire life be healthier. You will be pain-free, flexible and able to run, walk, skip, play tennis, shift fridges, play and generally have fun with life.

Move more exercise less [3]

If you are going to the gym three times a week don't fool yourself that you are fit. Movement is a daily activity and should include walking a minimum of 10,000 steps. As well as going to the gym, you need great posture and movement throughout your day. The gym does not tick your healthy activity box. In fact, treadmill running is counterproductive. It holds you in the same position for long periods of time, and that is the definition of RSI [repetitive strain injury], is it not?

Static gym machines are not ideal, unless of course you want to hang out with smelly teenagers or buff men (now there's a thought). Use free weights at home; the multiple loads and tensions on your body are much more beneficial to your shoulder and joint health. Static weights on a machine 'stress' your body in the same plane of movement – think RSI.

Back pain is 99.9% from bad posture

As a biomechanics instructor (that is, a Pilates teacher), I am staggered by the postures, aches, pains and debilitating deportment I see regularly.

An athletic runner – let's call her Amelia – stiffly shuffled into my class and explained that her colleagues ridiculed her posture. She felt she should do something. Rigid, in her mid-40s she had won several running competitions and was incredibly proud of her PBs (personal best running times). They were impressive. However, I couldn't help thinking: For how long? For how long are you going to be able to do this? Ligaments will snap, your hamstrings are going to push your hips out of place – you will suffer from backaches, misalignments, and undue stress and loads throughout your whole body.

During the course of the class, the stretches were too much for Amelia, sadly, and she didn't last more than a few terms. The movements were too painful, because her body had become used to running: one form of exercise in one plane of movement. Amelia's running career was successful, so why should she move through painful stretches? I could see her point, but my brain was screaming: Longevity! What are you going to be able to do five years from now?

Another interesting classmate is Henry, who came to my class in a similarly tight spot. His wife had encouraged, cajoled and shouted – and finally he arrived. The class loves Henry; he is an ex-footballer, with long legs, a great personality, and he's always willing to heckle from the back. He has stuck with Pilates and has improved miraculously. His body type is a 'back pain' classic: tall, long legs, long levers and played football all through his youth with no stretching. The Pilates moves are tough for him, but he has grit, determination and a lot of women watching. It does the trick.

Joseph Pilates and many of the original Pilates instructors were men, but men seem to suffer the most in class, to my amusement, I have to be honest. They sweat, swear and push and grunt because they use every muscle in their body, not just the one or two needed. Pilates is a slow flow activity, and is often referred to as 'the thinking person's exercise'. The strategy and focus in Pilates come from your inner working, and focused concentration on knowing which muscles are working. Concentration allows you to go deep and find your stabilising muscles and work on specific and isolated areas of your body. It strengthens your posterior chain, helping improve the daily function of your back.

General exercise, for want of a better word, works on the big levers, the big muscle groups close to the skin, which are called 'global muscles' or 'superficial muscles'. Your quads, six pack, pecs. The muscles that make you look good. Pilates, on the other hand, is interested in your internal muscles, the stabilisers that hold your body upright. To activate and strengthen your stabilisers, practise balancing on one leg. Plyometrics, which are exercises in which muscles exert maximum force in short intervals of time, such as pushing off quickly from the floor or equipment, are another great way to increase your dynamic balancing power.

TOP TIP

Wobbling on a balance board helps create strength – wobble more, get stronger.

Neutral spine throughout your day

Great balance and coordination come from endurance. Imagine that your back is held in place with guy ropes, as if you were pitching a tent, or visualise an electricity pylon with lots of strong legs to support the frame. [4]

The muscles of your back – your abdominal *(rectus abdominis)* at the front (six-pack), side abdominals (obliques), spinal erectors *(erector spinae)* – and your pelvis support your spine. They do this continuously. These muscles are stronger and act best when they are held in neutral position. Neutral spine is not flat to the floor. Try a flat back while standing up. What does that look like – natural? I think not. Neutral spine is the natural position of your spine when all three curves are present and in good alignment. It is vital to ensure that you can withstand loads whilst standing, sitting and walking throughout your normal day.

If you jar your back by stepping off a curb at a strange angle, your neutral spine will offset that load. The 'trauma' will reverberate right up your back, in a moment. Your natural curves can dissipate the load. Any imbalances in your body will immediately be brought to your attention when you jar your back: the force goes straight to the misalignment joint. If your hips are out of line with your shoulders, then *wham*, your hips will get the full force of the jarring.

Neutral spine means that your hips are lining up with your pubic bone. This will encourage a flat musculature structure, with your transverse abdominal muscle *(transversus abdominis)*, pubic bone and hips in alignment to your neutral lumbar spine – a natural lower back curve.

Your back needs to be worked in a pattern of endurance. Your muscles hold you upright for long periods of time, so your exercise needs to reflect this Too many open moves – similar to the 'up dog' back bends in yoga – are not comfortable for your back and can create hypermobility with excessive use. Your back performs better carrying out small, loaded, continuous movements. Little back lifts performed repeatedly with small loads create stability and strength. Large yoga 'up dog' flows create a wonderful openness to your spine, but muscle power and increased strength come from constant, low and loaded movements

The various parts of your body work in synergy, like an orchestra. The 'myofascial' physiotherapy and osteopathy gang that I hang out with believe that you have only one muscle – one muscle that covers your entire body – simply because all muscles are connected by myofascial, which is the dense, tough tissue bit. You see it clearly on a piece of raw chicken.

Some muscles work with several joints and if one joint is not functioning properly, that can constrain the movement of another joint. Osteopaths will tell you that pain in your right hip can affect the left shoulder or the left knee. Pain and destabilisation run diagonally back and forth across your body.

Limbs create movement and your hips and arms should be your prime movers. Pain arises when you use your back to make the moves. You see it all the time – a person hunching over a desk, a tall young woman trying to cover her body, computer use, bending from the middle of the back or the top of the back. It is so painful to watch, and it will cause extreme back issues in the future.

Create good movement patterns

Creating good movement patterns in your body, particularly for your back, is of vital importance. If you start the 0 to 5km or prepare for a half-marathon or start any exercise, be aware of doing too much too soon and causing injury.

I see it so often; it puts people off exercise for life. Create a good daily movement pattern, then start exercising. Don't start running if you have knocked knees, don't go for a commando challenge if your shoulders can't hold your own body weight.

Even athletes who have been running for a while need to mix it up a bit. Don't just run, or just practise yoga, Cross-fit, HIIT, or walk. Mix it up. Plateaus in your fitness, weight loss and your health occur when you do the same thing week in, week out. You need to participate in different types of exercise and movement. If you are working out in the same way, running the same mileage and doing the same class, you are no longer creating adaptations in your body. You may be reasonably fit within one discipline, but you have probably plateaued, are stalemate and no longer benefiting.

Good back strategies

Good back strategies include mixing and matching your movement and activities, doing three different types of exercise, to include muscular strength, cardiovascular and mind-body training. Add to this mindful movement every day, noticing how you walk and sit throughout the day. Avoid prolonged activity that includes sitting in one place for long periods of time. Your muscles and your connective tissue (myofascia) will get stiff and sore and start to impact on your muscles and joints.

Create movement from your hips

Hip hinges and shoulder work are essential to keeping your back strong. To avoid back injury, lift heavy objects close to your body line. Avoid twisting or jerking suddenly, obviously that isn't easy when you have a small wriggling child or dog. But generally, your back will benefit from stretching and twisting at regular intervals throughout the day so when you do have to work with a squirming, small 'lovely', your body can cope with the added stress of sudden jerky, movement. Hip hinging must be your movement default, moving from the hip and keeping your spine neutral. Move mindfully into this position, rather than hunching and lifting from the back. If you are feeling brave, ask your friends, family or me, "What is my posture like?"

About 20 years ago, Julie worked with me in the gym. We both taught aerobics, step and other crazy workouts. We both had one child and were trying to juggle tiredness, healthy eating, sanity and small children with school holidays. Luckily the gym we worked for had a kids' club, our sons met and played together. The boys played and did lots of exercise all day – it was all indoors and I have no idea how the supervisors coped with the noise in the huge gymnasium.

One day Julie turned up in tears. It was heartbreaking to witness. Her son had been diagnosed with severe curvature of the spine: kyphosis. Left untreated, it had progressed and had become chronic. The bones had begun to grow and set in that position, and it would take rehabilitation over a long time to realign the spine. I looked at her and said that I knew. Her response was, "Why on earth didn't you tell me?" I felt awful; I had assumed that she knew; I thought everyone could diagnose posture. I was timid, young(ish) and didn't speak up. The lesson I learned that day from Julie's pain and exasperation with me still haunts me.

Movement is the key to longevity, to a happy and healthy life. Biomechanically we should hang out of trees more often, which would encourage different loads being placed throughout your body. Sounds like fun!

Barefooted and free

Stretch your feet daily. I use a yoga mat under my feet each morning while making my beloved his tea.

I stretch my feet every morning because I run outside often. I love it. Being outside is a ritual I adore. It calms me, offers me peace, a calm space to order my thoughts. I love my cathedral of green and the bright spots of the blue sky. It is my version of blue-sky thinking.

The downside of this is that my calves are shot to pieces; my sports masseuse smiles with glee when she sees me. Calf massage is her favourite, my worst. Because I run so often, my calves have tightened up, but foot movement has helped to reduce this.

Similarly, because I teach Pilates so often my right psoas muscle is very tight. Fitness instructors aren't the fittest of specimens. We suffer from the same pitfalls of repetitive strain that office workers sitting in chairs do.

Female fitness instructors obsessed with lunges and squats while pregnant were 73.5% more likely to have pelvic floor dysfunction (I made that figure up, but the point is valid). After carrying three 10lb-babies and going through six pregnancies and three caesarean sections, exercising throughout, my pelvic floor should be at my ankles. You will be relieved to know that, after more than 20 years of teaching Pilates, I won't wee when I meet you. My pelvic floor is great, but I still don't trust a trampoline.

Weightlifting should not be done in the same shoes you run in. Lifting weights exerts a lot of pressure on your feet and ligaments. Running shoes are generally elevated at the back and your hips are then pushed forward of your pubic bone – you won't be able to lift in alignment. Big secret, big reveal: I lift weights barefooted. I allow my feet to find my balance and balance the load through my legs and feet.

You must find your sticky spots

Myofascial release and barefoot running were very trendy. Barefoot running has its place, but not for a modern western girl. Zola Budd, the South African-born girl who competed for Great Britain in the 1984 Olympics, had been running barefoot all her life, as had her local competitors. Feet need to create very big callus to adapt to this type of running. Most of us have been wearing 'toddler shoes' from birth, our heels slight raised, our hips slightly tipped forward. Therefore, adapting away from these musculature imprints and running barefoot will damage our feet, knees and Achilles tendons. Your tendons will take the brunt of the transformation to barefoot running.

Barefoot running is incredibly difficult and arduous to adapt to, but barefoot walking is very accessible for all.

Assessing your gait, however, is also something we can all do. If your knees are knocking, your calves killing you or your hips are painful, then a running shop or Pilates instructor can assess your gait. Find running shoes that will aid your gait, and ensure that you buy good trainers, regularly.

I have lots of trainers. I have posh trainers for going out in, running trainers that are comfortable, blue trainers that I bought but are too high and stay in my cupboard. I like to swap my trainers – new to old, different types so that I mix it up.

Look for your tight spots

Inflammation of the kind that causes heel pain (*plantar fasciitis*) can flare up anywhere in your body. Inflammation in your shoulder will create frozen shoulder or tennis elbow. Our plane of movement has become very limited – even if we wanted to, sadly, we don't hang from trees enough. Our typical movements tend to revolve around typing on a keyboard, sitting with rounded shoulders or being slumped on the settee. Our movement is far more restricted, with minimal variations in the force and loads applied to your joints. This tends to lead to aches and pains that can be debilitating.

Preventative biomechanics mean using your shoulders and hips in varying different ways, not just squats and lunges or typing and sitting.

Tight spots are clues to your body's internal health. Your feet are one place to look, your shoulders and of course your back are others. Bad posture creates these little 'sticky' spots where your myofascia has got stuck, when your cells stick together and create barriers to blood flow, preventing nutrients from accessing those sites. The lack of blood flow will affect your overall body immunity.

Posture alignment and myofascial release are in my blogs on my Get Gorgeous site under 'exercise' at www. get-gorgeous.com/blogs. There is plenty of specific information there to help you get started with myofascial release, Pilates and great posture. I post weekly vlogs and Pilates workouts on the site and on my YouTube channel: Adele's Pilates.

Forest bathing

Perhaps I haven't convinced you to get up at 6am and go running in the rain, but how about forest bathing? Getting outside is going to do more for your health than three times a week in the gym. Moving your arms vigorously and walking over uneven surfaces is going to create a stronger, more varied muscle pattern for your body.

Forest bathing and walking among the trees create a calming effect within you. Your nervous system adapts and slows, and you reduce your production of cortisol, the stress hormone. Walking in your cathedral of green will reduce stress, anxiety and anger. The exercise itself will help resolve insomnia and improve your mental clarity. Trees release chemicals, called phytoncides, which research has found to boost your immune system. Being surrounded by greenery is important. Green light is life-affirming and pleasing, while blue light, as we discussed, wakes you up when you are trying to go to sleep. Furthermore, the difference between light and shade contributes to your sense of being alive and your connection to nature.

Mindful movement daily

Walking daily, a minimum of 10,000 steps, is imperative. A free challenge that I promote on my Get Gorgeous website at get-gorgeous.com/healthy-tools includes daily videos and helpful hints and tips about walking well and motivation to keep going.

Bad posture and tight muscles mean that walking can become a kind of falling forward, whereas great walking technique will aid your stability and posture. Good posture keeps energy circulating in your body. Bad posture is exhausting and drains you. Bad posture will keep your energy low and lead to low-level tiredness.

Movement is essential for your heart

Your heart can't do all the work. While your heart is amazing and pumps blood round your body, movement helps your heart function. Your arteries pump the blood around your body and assist your heart. Moving is the answer to a healthy heart. Pumping movement or simply swinging your arms is going to assist your heart function.

Great walking posture

Swinging your arms will loosen your shoulders after hours of prolonged, stationary activity at a desk. It will warm them up and help to unlock your shoulders. Push off your back foot, create a spring action with your feet and lightly stiffen or brace your abdominals to create a support for your back. A short burst of speed walking is a simple HIIT [high-intensity interval training] workout and can form part of a dynamic fartlek training session (the word causes great amusement to my 'teenage' husband). Fartlek is not farting all the way round the woods, but simply mixing periods of slower running with short bursts of interval sessions. It originated in Sweden – the word means 'speed play' in Swedish – and offers you a varied workout that will enable you to use different energy sources in your body for fuel. Which leads me on cleverly to fuel for exercise.

Which body type do you have?

Are you an ectomorph, endomorph or mesomorph? All members of the Tony Hart's *Take Hart* Morph family. I fancy myself as a mesomorph, strong and athletic, but with my booty, maybe not. An ectomorph needs to eat differently from a mesomorph.

This kind of detail will become apparent to you when you start noticing how you feel around food, during the day and how you fast. The way you exercise and your response to glucose will all be affected by your body type. Interestingly, there are body-type diets you can follow, or you could simply look at your own body and spend some time owning your body, understanding it better, which will serve you better in the long run.

Mesomorphs like Venus Williams (the tennis player), and Halle Berry, Madonna and Jessica Alba are strong and athletic. You can see why I want to be in this group. Ectomorphs like Gwyneth Paltrow, Kate Moss and Cameron Diaz can tolerate a lot of carbs: in fact, they need carbs and therefore glucose to feel energised, and are going to struggle with an intermittent fasting schedule. That body type works better with carbs. Endomorphs like mesomorphs can get on with fewer carbs. Endomorphs are people like Kim Kardashian, Beyoncé and Jennifer Lopez, who have a high fat to muscle ratio, with a beautiful round body shape and hold excess fat on their hips.

Balancing macros with movement

Women react very differently from men when it comes to stress, fasting, exercise performance and food intake. Women's bodies do not like to go hungry. You have probably experienced that your body will hold on to fat for the sake of your potential children – whether you have had them or not. Women's bodies are geared for producing offspring. Athletes who work out excessively or gym bunnies with body dysmorphia are in danger of upsetting their hormone balance (resulting in no periods), but high stress can also create the same unfavourable body balance for your hormones.

The hypothalamic-pituitary- adrenal (HPA) axis is a major neuroendocrine system that controls reactions to stress and regulates many body processes, including digestion, sexuality, and energy storage and expenditure. It has a strong influence on factors involved in the balance and regulation of your metabolism, which can lead to periods stopping and metabolic stress when there is perceived starvation.

Exercise, like life, can create stress for your body, which will affect your mood, your digestion, your libido and your immune system. The pituitary gland, which produces and secretes growth hormone (remember him, how useful he is with muscle strength and stimulating cell growth as we age), also stimulates thyroid function. The female thyroid is very delicate, while the man's behaves more like a brick. Therefore you need to treat your body with respect, listening to it intuitively and finding a healthy nutrition pathway that suits you.

As a guide, I would suggest strength training a couple of times a week with free weights and consuming more carbohydrates such as quinoa (has lots of protein and is a seed rather than a grain), berries and potatoes after exercise – I do love potatoes! But keep these 'treasures' until after you have exercised when the glucose from the carbohydrate is required to push protein into the muscle and create stronger muscles.

Insulin, testosterone and growth hormone are anabolic hormones, which means that they synthesise, for example, creating stronger bone mass, muscle mass, reproductive organs and skin. Insulin and carbohydrates are important for your diet, your health and your weight loss, however you do need to pay attention to when you eat them.

Carb cycling and exercise

On your HIIT and low-intensity (slow run) days, eat fewer carbs. If you are eating salad and fish or other protein for lunch, and eggs for breakfast, you will be amazed at how few carbs you are actually eating.

When you are going for longer duration and harder intensity workouts, enjoy more carbs, including the starchy variety. Green carbs should be eaten at every meal (by green I mean vegetables, not just leafy salad).

Carb intake should be varied according to the body types that I mentioned earlier. An endomorph like Jennifer Lopez will require fewer carbs and ectomorphs like Cameron Diaz will need much more. A mesomorph like Halle Berry should consume around 40% of her calories as carbs, or less. I eat this proportion of carbs only when I am exercising hard and fast (which isn't that often). You will find your 'carb' sweet spot.

As discussed previously, if you are really interested in tracking your consumption of macronutrients, download the *My Fitness Pal* app. I tracked my percentages for a while and it helped me see my relative intake of fats, protein and carbs. I eat salmon, mackerel, cheese, nuts and avocado, which means my omega-3 fat levels are high.

Research found that low-carb diets burned the most calories and the biggest improvement in insulin sensitivity:[5]

- Low-fat diet: 60% carbs, 20% fats 20% protein

- Low-glycaemic-index diet: 40% carbs, 40% fats, 20% protein

- Low-carb diet: 10% carbs, 60% fats, 30% protein

Finding what works for you takes patience and time, listening to your inner intuition and working with a professional will help you to find your perfect carb balance. This in turn will improve your body composition, your health and optimise your training and movement strategies.

Before you go…

Water and exercise

Water will flush out toxins and prevent headaches, boost your immune system, improve your complexion, and increase your brain power and energy. It will aid and maintain digestive regularity, help you to regulate body temperature, prevent bad breath and improve your heart health.

Water helps to dilute your blood and enables it to flow through your body. Glycated haemoglobin is made when the glucose in your body can't be used properly, so more of it sticks to your red blood cells and builds up in your blood, which can damage your blood vessels. Water helps to thin the blood, reduce this viscosity and make it less likely to clot and cause blockages.

Water is essential when you are doing any type of fasting, whether it is 12:12 or 5:2 or something stricter. Staying hydrated is essential. If you want to increase your water intake, join me for the water challenge by visiting my website at www.get-gorgeous.com/healthy-tools/

Balance your electrolytes

If you feel that you suffer regularly from heat cramps, muscle cramps or headaches, you may consider adding electrolytes to your water. Electrolytes include sodium, potassium, calcium, magnesium and other essential minerals. While many people are reducing their sodium intake, they are not increasing the potassium in their diets. Potassium is an electrolyte that conducts nerve impulses and muscle contractions, regulates the flow of fluids and nutrients into and out of your body cells. Sodium raises your blood pressure, while potassium lowers it. The body works best when the ratio between sodium and potassium is just right – a lower sodium-potassium ratio may help to keep the bones stronger, reduce the burden on the kidneys and improve cardiovascular health. Processed foods unfortunately have a huge amount of salt (sodium), while many fruits and vegetables are excellent sources of potassium but contain little sodium.

TOP TIP

Swapping out heavily processed foods in favour of nutrient-dense whole foods will automatically lower your sodium intake and increase your consumption of potassium.

Avoid synthetic calories

Water and exercise are key. Over the years, I have tried fizz sticks, isotonic drinks, fruit juices and shakes. You simply don't need them: stick to water. We discussed fructose in the nutrition chapter, and I mention it again here in the context of the synthetic fructose found in high-fructose corn sugar (HFCS), which is deadly. HFCS is found in most fizzy drinks, including your so-called healthy and cleverly packaged elderflower cordial. It is also used in low-fat yoghurt, sports drinks (such as Gatorade) and bottled tea. Aspartame, which is used as a sugar substitute in thousands of food and drink products, including zero-calorie drinks, is another synthetic product best avoided.

Include green tea

I drink a lot of green tea. It took me a while to become accustomed to it, but now I drink it easily. In fact, one of the Get Gorgeous principles is drink green tea, because it is packed with antioxidants. The flavonoids in green tea means that it can increase your metabolism and reduce those hippy free radicals that are so damaging for your body.

Conclusion

While sipping my green tea, I have to ask, what are you excited to pick up and run with now? I am interested; are you going to talk to yourself more often and question why you thought or said that? Out loud and proud? Are you going to remove all gluten from your diet starting from today? I thought not. Perhaps you can start by ditching cereal and worry a little less about what milk to put in your tea and instead notice how much protein you are adding to your meals. Worry less about the micro and look more to the macro. I know you will never look at a green smoothie the same way or a healthy, packaged goggy goggy bean bar (that is a made-up bean, by the way).

Perhaps you will attend your first Pilates class, or follow me on YouTube, knowing that Pilates will help you live a long and healthy life in a strong and adaptable body.

Open your mind, open your heart and put yourself first. This may feel alien and uncomfortable, but by pushing yourself to the limits of your comfort zone you will notice the change. It will be slow at first.

My purpose with this book is to begin that change. As coaches, we are asked to explore our own personal and business core values, what we bring to clients. A client taught me mine: she explained that I was down to earth, genuine, that I worked with integrity and sincerity, and she felt that I had my finger on the nutritional pulse.

Nutritionists and psychotherapists have said that this book may be too complicated, too much. I wanted to keep to my core values and make nutrition easy. While I have mentioned several emerging concepts in this book, the theme is simple: get out of your own way and eat a farmhouse diet – more veg, proteins and fats and fewer processed carbs. 'Intermittent fasting' is a posh way of saying 'delay your breakfast' and 'carb cycling' simply means eating more carbs on the days you exercise really hard. Your posture is far more important than how many times you go to the gym. Your body is perfect, your body is gorgeous; listen to your body more and your mind less.

You have got this covered, gorgeous; tell Horace and Rose to sit quietly.

What's next?

1. Register your book online at get-gorgeous.com/book-registration or simply scan the QR code at the back of this book. You will receive my free 'fat chart', 'know your why' and I'll throw in some Pilates workouts to get you started with great posture.

2. Join my free water or walking challenge www.get-gorgeous.com/healthy-tools

3. Join my online 10-day Pilates based tummy challenge on my gorgeous website www.get-gorgeous.com/healthy-tools

4. Discover more about Pilates on my YouTube channel search on YouTube for 'Adele's Pilates' or for more in-depth Pilates visit my Pilates website www.adelespilates.co.uk/online

5. If you would like more support, apply for a one-to-one coaching session via my website: www.get-gorgeous.com. I am more than prepared to offer

my 50% of the discussion; I will arrive with an open heart, and if you do the same your results will be transformational.

References

Introduction

(1)   Wikipedia (nd). Starvation response. [online] https://en.wikipedia.org/wiki/Starvation_response

Chapter 1

(1)   Wessels Living History Farm website (nd). Farming in the 1930s. [online] https://livinghistoryfarm. org/farminginthe30s/life_04.html

(2)   British Nutrition Foundation website (nd). How the war changed nutrition: from there to now. [online] https://www.nutrition.org.uk/nutritioninthenews/ wartimefood/warnutrition.html

(3)   Lamberton J (2017). *Big Ideas… For Small Businesses: Simple Practical Tools and Tactics to Help Small Business Grow.*

(4)   Cialdini RB (2007). *Influence: The Psychology of Persuasion.*

(5)   Dweck CS (2012). *Mindset: How You Can Fulfil Your Potential.* New York: Constable & Robinson.

(6)   McDermott I and Jago W (2001). *The NLP Coach: A Comprehensive Guide to Personal Well-Being and Professional Success.* London: Piatkus Books.

(7)   Olson J (2005). *The Slight Edge: Turning Simple Disciplines into Massive Success & Happiness* – 8th Anniversary edition.

(8)   Brown M (2008). *Alchemy of the Heart: Transform Turmoil into Peace Through Emotional Integration.* Newburyport, Massachusetts: Hampton Roads Publishing Company.

(9)   Ravikant K (2012). *Love Yourself Like Your Life Depends on It.* CreateSpace Independent Publishing Platform.

(10)   Hall K (2010). *Aspire: Discovering Your Purpose Through the Power of Words.* William Morrow.

(11)   Rubin G (2016). *Better Than Before: What I Learned About Making and Breaking Habits – to Sleep More, Quit Sugar, Procrastinate Less, and Generally Build a Happier Life.* Two Roads.

(12)   Zander LH (2017). *Maybe It's You: Cut the Crap. Face Your Fears. Love Your Life.* Hachette Books.

(13)   Ditzler J (2006). *Your Best Year Yet! A Proven Method for Making the Next 12 Months Your Most Successful Ever: Make the Next 12 Months Your Best Ever!* Harper Element.

(14)   Ferguson C (nd). *A Stealthy Way to Beat Procrastination.* [blog] https://carolineferguson.com/stealthy-way-beat-procrastination/

(15)   Mohr T (2014). *Playing Big: Find Your Voice, Your Mission, Your Message.* Gotham Books.

(16)   Sineck S (2011). *Start with Why: How Great Leaders Inspire Everyone to Take Action.* Penguin.

(17)   Olson J (2005). *The Slight Edge: Turning Simple Disciplines Into Massive Success & Happiness* – 8th anniversary edition.

Chapter 2

(1) Peters S (2012). *The Chimp Paradox: The Mind Management Programme to Help You Achieve Success, Confidence and Happiness*. Vermilion.

(2) Stickland A (nd). *Aerobics gear improves confidence.* [blog] https://get-gorgeous.com/active-wear-worth-wear/

(3) Peters S (2012). *The Chimp Paradox: The Mind Management Programme to Help You Achieve Success, Confidence and Happiness*. Vermilion.

(4) Draganescu A (nd). *Maslow's pyramid is about scarcity and privilege.* [blog] https://medium.com/@andraganescu/maslow-s-pyramid-is-about-scarcity-and-privilege-ea742f085d60

(5) Jones A (2018, 1 October). *I was on a diet for 18 years. Here's what I learned …* [online] https://www.bbc.co.uk/bbcthree/article/6b0548de-903f-4b15-8dd8-5c11bed79efc

(6) McDermott I and Jago W (2001). *The NLP Coach: A Comprehensive Guide to Personal Well-Being and Professional Success*. London: Piatkus Books.

(7) Heath C and Heath D (2011). *Switch: How to change things when change is hard* (pp28–32). Random House Business.

(8) Hardy D (2011). *The Compound Effect: Jumpstart Your Income, Your Life, Your Success*. Carroll & Graf.

Chapter 3

(1)   Nelson SK, Layous K, Cole SW and Lyubomirsky S (2016). Do unto others or treat yourself? The effects of prosocial and self-focused behavior on psychological flourishing. *Emotion, 16*(6), (pp 850–861). http://psycnet. apa.org/record/2016-19956-001

(2)   Ruiz DM (2018). *The Four Agreements: Practical Guide to Personal Freedom.* Amber-Allen Publishing.

(3)   The pursuit of happiness. [website] http://www. pursuit-of-happiness.org/science-of-happiness/

(4)   Achor S (2011). *The Happiness Advantage: The Seven Principles of Positive Psychology that Fuel Success and Performance at Work* (p42).

(5)   Achor S (2011). *The Happiness Advantage: The Seven Principles of Positive Psychology that Fuel Success and Performance at Work* (pp47–58).

(6)   Achor S (2011). *The Happiness Advantage: The Seven Principles of Positive Psychology that Fuel Success and Performance at Work* (p92).

(7)   Achor S (2011). *The Happiness Advantage: The Seven Principles of Positive Psychology that Fuel Success and Performance at Work* Gorilla experiment (pp95–98).

(8)   Achor S (2011). *The Happiness Advantage: The Seven Principles of Positive Psychology that Fuel Success and Performance at Work* Wiseman experiment (pp98-99).

(9)   The Balanced WorkLife Company (2017, 15 March). *What Marshmallows Can Teach You About Emotional Intelligence.* [online] https://balancedworklife.com/ emotional-intelligence-marshmallow/

(10)   Achor S (2011). *The Happiness Advantage: The Seven Principles of Positive Psychology that Fuel Success and Performance at Work* Maid Experiment (pp73-74).

(11)   Achor S (2011). *The Happiness Advantage: The Seven Principles of Positive Psychology that Fuel Success and Performance at Work* (p109).

(12)   Vale J (2011). *Kick the Drink … Easily!* Crown House Publishing.

(13)   Adlaf EW et al, University of Alabama (2017, 30 January). *Adult-born neurons modify excitatory synaptic transmission to existing neurons.* [online] https://elifesciences.org/articles/19886

(14)   Achor S (2011). *The Happiness Advantage: The Seven Principles of Positive Psychology that Fuel Success and Performance at Work* (pp136–137).

(15)   Zander RS and Zander B (2000). *The Art of Possibility: Transforming Professional and Personal Life.* Harvard Business Review Press.

Chapter 4

(1)   Hamilton DR (2008). *How Your Mind Can Heal Your Body.* Hay House UK.

(2)   Gage FH (2002). Neurogenesis in the Adult Brain. *Journal of Neuroscience, 22*(3), (pp612–613). www.jneurosci.org/content/22/3/612

(3)   Brazier Y (2018). *What are stem cells, and what do they do?* [online] https://www.medicalnewstoday.com/articles/323343.php

(4)   Peters S (2012). *The Chimp Paradox: The Mind Management Programme to Help You Achieve Success, Confidence and Happiness.* Vermilion.

(5)   Heath C and Heath D (2011). *Switch: How to change things when change is hard.* Random House Business.

(6)   Lamberton J (2017). *Big Ideas… For Small Businesses: Simple Practical Tools and Tactics to Help Small Business Grow.*

Chapter 5

(1)   Brown M (2008). *Alchemy of the Heart: Transform Turmoil into Peace Through Emotional Integration.* Newburyport, Massachusetts: Hampton Roads Publishing Company.

(2)   Brown M (2008). *Alchemy of the Heart: Transform Turmoil into Peace Through Emotional Integration.* Newburyport, Massachusetts: Hampton Roads Publishing Company.

(3)   Bernstein G (2014). *Miracles Now: 108 Life-Changing Tools for Less Stress, More Flow and Finding Your True Purpose.* Hay House UK.

(4)   James V (2018). On boredom. *CAM (Cambridge Alumni Magazine), 84.* [online] https://www.cam.ac.uk/cammagazine/benefitsofboredom

(5)   James V (2018). On boredom. *CAM (Cambridge Alumni Magazine), 84.* [online] https://www.cam.ac.uk/cammagazine/benefitsofboredom

Chapter 6

(1)   Stickland A. *How to add vegetarian protein into your healthy diet.* [blog] https://get-gorgeous.com/add-vegetarian-protein-healthy-diet/

(2)   Perlmutter D (2014). *Grain Brain: The Surprising Truth about Wheat, Carbs, and Sugar – Your Brain's Silent Killers* (p74).

(3)   P. Barberger-Gateua, et al 'Dietary Patterns and Risk of Dementia: The three city Cohort study' Neurology 69 no 20 (Nov 13 2007) (1921-30).

(4)   Teicholz N (2014). *The Big Fat Surprise: Why Butter, Meat and Cheese Belong in a Healthy Diet*, (p14).

(5)   UK Stats on obesity – https://www.england.nhs.uk/2014/09/serious-about-obesity/ https://en.wikipedia.org/wiki/Obesity_in_the_United_Kingdom

(6)   Perlmutter D (2014). *Grain Brain: The Surprising Truth about Wheat, Carbs, and Sugar – Your Brain's Silent Killers*

(7)   Teicholz N (2014). The Big Fat Surprise: why butter, meat, and cheese belong in a healthy diet.

(8)   BBC. *Rationing: Could the WW2 diet make you healthier?* [online] www.bbc.co.uk/guides/zqftn39

(9)   Van Berge-Henegouwen GP and Mulder CJ (1993). Pioneers in the gluten free diet: Willem-Karel Dicke 1905-1962, over 50 years of gluten free diet. Gut, 34(11), (pp1473–5). https://www.ncbi.nlm.nih.gov/pmc/articles/PMC1374403/

(10)   Perlmutter D (2014). *Grain Brain: The Surprising Truth about Wheat, Carbs, and Sugar – Your Brain's Silent Killers* (p62).

(11)   Taubes G (2012). *Why We Get Fat*. Anchor Books.

(12)   https://www.sevencountriesstudy.com/about-

the-study/

(13)   Yudkin J (2012). *Pure, White and Deadly: How Sugar Is Killing Us and What We Can Do to Stop It.* Penguin.

(14)   https://www.telegraph.co.uk/health-fitness/nutrition/52-author-michael-mosley-im-proof-low-fat-diets-dont-work/

(15)   The American Journal of Clinical Nutrition (online) Saturated fat, carbohydrate, and cardiovascular disease.
Patty W Siri-Tarino Qi Sun Frank B Hu Ronald M Krauss Volume 91, Issue 3, 1 March 2010, Pages 502–509, https://doi.org/10.3945/ajcn.2008.26285 https://academic.oup.com/ajcn/article/91/3/502/4597078

(16)   Perlmutter D (2014). *Grain Brain: The Surprising Truth about Wheat, Carbs, and Sugar – Your Brain's Silent Killers* page 81 smoking is endorsed same kind of ignorance.

(17)   Perlmutter D (2014). *Grain Brain: The Surprising Truth about Wheat, Carbs, and Sugar – Your Brain's Silent Killers* (p86) diabetes exploded 1997-2007.

(18)   Kendrick M (2008). *The Great Cholesterol Con.* John Blake Publishing Ltd (p58).

(19)   Stickland A. "Coconut Oil is pure poison" headlines to TERRIFY! [blog] https://get-gorgeous.com/coconut-oil-is-pure-poison-headlines-to-terrify/

(20)   Taubes G (2001, 30 march). The Soft Science of Dietary Fat. Science, 291(5513), (2536-2556).

(21)   Perlmutter D (2014). *Grain Brain: The Surprising Truth about Wheat, Carbs, and Sugar – Your Brain's Silent Killers.*

(22)   Campbell TC and Campbell TM (2006). *The China Study: The Most Comprehensive Study of Nutrition Ever Conducted and the Startling Implications for Diet, Weight Loss and Long-Term Health.*

(23)   Minger D. *The China Study: Fact or Fallacy?* [online] https://deniseminger.com/2010/07/07/the-china-study-fact-or-fallac/(online) (pp160–164).

(24)   Diamond J (1997) Guns, Germs & Steel A short history of everybody for the last 13,000 years.

(25)   Davis W (2011). *Wheat Belly: Lose the Wheat, Lose the Weight, and Find Your Path Back to Health.* Emmaus, Penn: Rodale.

(26)   Kendrick M (2008). *The Great Cholesterol Con.* John Blake Publishing Ltd.

(27)   Kendrick M (2008). *The Great Cholesterol Con.* John Blake Publishing Ltd.

(28)   Perlmutter D (2014). *Grain Brain: The Surprising Truth about Wheat, Carbs, and Sugar – Your Brain's Silent Killers* (p63) bread gives you a buzz.

(29)   Perlmutter D (2014). *Grain Brain: The Surprising Truth about Wheat, Carbs, and Sugar – Your Brain's Silent Killers.*

(30)   Perlmutter D (2014). *Grain Brain: The Surprising Truth about Wheat, Carbs, and Sugar – Your Brain's Silent Killers* (p210) the fatter you are the smaller the brain.

(31)   Stickland A. *STOP drinking probiotic drinks!* [blog] https://get-gorgeous.com/stop-drinking-probiotic-drinks/

(32)   Stickland A. *Is not enough gut bacteria making you fat?* [blog] https://get-gorgeous.com/is-not-enough-gut-bacteria-making-you-fat/

(33)   Perlmutter D (2014). *Grain Brain: The Surprising Truth about Wheat, Carbs, and Sugar – Your Brain's Silent Killers.*

(34)   Enders G, Enders J and Shaw D (2015). Gut: The Inside Story of our Body's Most Underrated Organ. Vancouver: Greystone Books.

(35)   Enders G, Enders J and Shaw D (2015). Gut: The Inside Story of our Body's Most Underrated Organ. Vancouver: Greystone Books.

(36)   Hamilton A (2014). *Eat Fast Slim: The Life-Changing Fasting Diet for Amazing Weight Loss and Optimum Health.* Watkins Publishing.

(37)   Hamilton A (2014). Eat Fast Slim: The Life-Changing Fasting Diet for Amazing Weight Loss and Optimum Health. Watkins Publishing.

(38)   Woodgate M. *The AMAZING Health Benefits of Intermittent Fasting.* [online] https://www.bodyblueprint.co.nz/the-amazing-health-benefits-of-intermittent-fasting/

Chapter 7

(1)   Aronson D (2009). Cortisol – its role in stress, inflammation, and indications for diet therapy. *Today's Dietitian, 11*(11), pp38–41.

(2)   Hamilton A Eat Fast Slim The Life-Changing Fasting Diet for Amazing Loss and Optimum Health (2013).

(3)   Jamieson S (2017, 2 July). Fish becoming transgender from contraceptive pill chemicals being flushed down household drains. *The Telegraph*. [online] www.telegraph.co.uk/news/2017/07/02/fish-becoming-transgender-contraceptive-pill-chemicals-flushed/

(4)   Stickland A Menopausal weight sits on your TUMMY – does that have to be true? (blog) https://get-gorgeous.com/menopausal-weight-sits-tummy-true/

(5)   Dr Eric Berg Estrogen, mood & Menopause Youtube: https://www.youtube.com/watch?v=6vn7-OjX4Kc

(6)   Kendrick M (2008). *The Great Cholesterol Con*. John Blake Publishing Ltd (p102).

(7)   Rossouw JE (2000). Debate: The potential role of estrogen in the prevention of heart disease in women after menopause. *Current controlled trials in cardiovascular medicine*, *1*(3), pp135-138.   https://www.ncbi.nlm.nih.gov/pmc/articles/PMC59619/

(8)   Kendrick M (2008). *The Great Cholesterol Con*. John Blake Publishing Ltd (p105).

(9)   Kendrick M (2008). *The Great Cholesterol Con*. John Blake Publishing Ltd (pp238-243).

(10)   Kendrick M (2008). *The Great Cholesterol Con*. John Blake Publishing Ltd 14 Country Study (pp74-75).

Chapter 8

(1)   C. W. Cotman, et al "Exercise Builds Brain Health: Key Roles of Growth Factor Cascades and

inflation," Trends in Neuroscience 30, no. 9 (September 2007) (pp464-72).

(2)   Liu CJ and Latham NK (2009). Progressive resistance strength training for improving physical function in older adults. *The Cochrane database of systematic reviews*, (3), CD002759. doi:10.1002/14651858.CD002759.pub2.

(3)   Bowman K. *Move your DNA: Restore Your Health Through Natural Movement.*

(4)   McGill S (2015). *Back Mechanic.* Backfitpro Inc.

(5)   Ebbeling CB, Swain JF, Feldman HA, et al (2012). Effects of Dietary Composition on Energy Expenditure During Weight-Loss Maintenance. *JAMA*, *307*(24), (2627–2634). doi:10.1001/jama.2012.6607

Join my community of like-minded gorgeous girls

Like-minded people are the secret to your gorgeous success. It is important to surround yourself with harmonious, confident women who will support and nurture you.

If you would love to feel supported and support others in our gorgeous journey together simply search for adelegetgorgeous on Facebook or join me on other social platforms:

in LinkedIn: www.linkedin.com/in/adelestickland

f Facebook: www.facebook.com/adelegetgorgeous

🐦 Twitter: www.twitter.com/adelestickland

📷 Instagram: www.instagram.com/adele_stickland

P Pinterest: www.pinterest.co.uk/adelegetgorgeous/

YouTube Youtube: Adele's Pilates

What others say about working with Adele

"I found Adele to be warm, sincere with great integrity. Adele opened the space for me to communicate, held that space and continually checked to see where I was emotionally. I would highly recommend working with Adele as an NLP master practitioner, life coach and hypnotherapist.. You feel listened to, supported and cared for!"

Teresa Reay, director, Evolve Marketing

"I found Adele to be a superb personal coach; she is someone I trust personally and professionally to support me into wellbeing, particularly when I've lost my way in supporting myself. Adele coached me to draw on my strength and self-esteem during a period of great personal challenge and stress. I needed to continue to lead and hold space for others who were more vulnerable and realised on meeting her that I had lost myself in the process. Adele cleanly moved me through my inner resistance to taking care of myself without me realising I had acted – it was quite spooky. She made me feel human and real again and created a process of change that felt accessible and possible."

Jennifer Parry, leadership coach to CEOs

"Adele is the MOST AMAZING WOMAN and incredible health coach that anyone can choose to work with!"

Shelley Hutchinson, business coach

"I can highly recommend working with Adele for health, fitness, and weight-loss issues. Her advice is clear, practical, and simple to follow, and what she doesn't know about health and nutrition probably isn't worth knowing! With her kind and caring nature and approach, she is always in your corner to give support. Give her a call; you won't go far wrong."

Kate Thorpe, stress therapist and coach

"Adele is a wealth of information, experience, expertise and wisdom in the field of women's health for the over 40s. She is also an absolute joy to work with and be around. So much positive energy, fun, authenticity. She really cares about her clients and the value she adds. I totally recommend her."

Mandy Mucklat, executive coach for leaders

Register your book

Join the Gorgeous Girls and register your book to receive current health tips and Pilates exercises and more. You'll be added to my mailing list to receive weekly health updates and be the first to know about my Pilates retreats, home and abroad.

Simply scan the QR code below or visit
https://www.get-gorgeous.com/book-registration

About the author

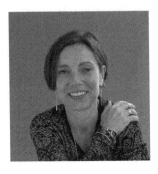

Adele Stickland, mum of three, is the founder of Get Gorgeous, an online platform dedicated to inspiring and empowering women to have great health.

While working in an ambitious and stressful full-time job, Adele juggled keeping herself safe and nurtured while caring for her family. After a decade of infertility, she crashed out and pursued her passion in health and Pilates. She has educated hundreds of women on the role of nutrition, movement and having a healthy mindset. She has worked in the health industry for 20 years.

Her website and blogs reach hundreds of people every month, and hundreds more attend her live Pilates classes, workshops and retreats.

A powerful combination of personal experience and industry background means that Adele is ideally placed to understand the needs of women looking for solace in their minds and gorgeous bodies.